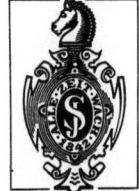

Clinical Practice in Urology
Series Editor: Geoffrey D. Chisholm

Urinary Diversion

Edited by
Michael Handley Ashken

With 53 Figures

Springer-Verlag
Berlin Heidelberg New York 1982

Michael Handley Ashken, BSc, MS, FRCS

Consultant Urologist
Norfolk and Norwich Hospital
Norwich, Norfolk, England

Series Editor
Geoffrey D. Chisholm, FRCS
Professor of Surgery,
University of Edinburgh,
Scotland

ISBN-13: 978-1-4471-1322-5   e-ISBN-13: 978-1-4471-1320-1
DOI: 10.1007/978-1-4471-1320-1

Library of Congress Cataloging in Publication Data
Urinary Diversion. (Clinical practice in urology) Bibliography: p. Includes index.
1. Urinary organs — Surgery. 2. Urinary diversion.
I. Ashken, Michael Handley, 1931– . II. Series. [DNLM: 1. Urinary Diversion
WJ 168 U73] RD578.U74 617'.461 82-826
ISBN 0-387-11273-1 (U.S.) AACR2

Filmset and printed by Spottiswoode Ballantyne Ltd, Colchester, Essex

2128/3916-543210

Series Editor's Foreword

Such an important subject as urinary diversion is unlikely to remain unchanged and unchallenged for long. The problem is to determine when is an appropriate time to examine current clinical practice of this major urological procedure.

Historically, urinary diversion began with attempts to resolve the distressing problems associated with ectopia vesicae; later, urinary diversion was extended to help those patients with neurological problems of bladder function and with malignant diseases of the lower urinary tract. A significant landmark in the development and use of these procedures came with the introduction of a uretero-ileostomy (ileal conduit) by Bricker. With this diversion, faecal and urinary streams were separated and the incidence of metabolic and infective problems dramatically reduced. The procedure was received with great enthusiasm and indeed the pendulum soon swung so far in its favour that some urologists would scarcely admit to carrying out an occasional ureterosigmoidostomy.

The impact of change in a surgical technique can be slow to determine especially when, numerically, it is an uncommon procedure and when the follow-up is hoped to match normal life expectancy. Thus the impact of ileal conduits has taken some years to evaluate and only during the past decade have the data been sufficient to show the advantages and disadvantages.

This book is a landmark in the literature on this subject. The editor has selected eminent contributors who have described the main clinical groups where urinary diversion is an important aspect of management. Each contributor has produced a scholarly, authoritative essay evaluating the subject. These, together with a chapter on stoma care and a discourse on the present status of urinary reservoirs, all add up to a most comprehensive text on the clinical practice of urinary diversion.

The reader can be assured of good practical advice and guidance, for this is the purpose of the series. Mr. Ashken can be confident that he and his colleagues have achieved a standard of style that will have great attraction for those who seek 'continuing medical education'. I anticipate that this book in this new series will be keenly welcomed by all urologists.

Edinburgh, January 1982   Geoffrey Chisholm

Preface

This volume aims to review our present thoughts on Urinary Diversion, emphasising the wide range of both conservative and operative procedures available for the treatment of any individual patient. The requirements will vary enormously depending on a number of factors such as age, sex, intelligence, build, the disease process and its prognosis and their socio-economic environment. The abilities and expectations of our patients will cover a wide spectrum of life.

To recommend a urinary diversion must rank amongst the most major of decisions in any surgical practice. In the younger age group, urinary diversion is most commonly done to maintain or improve deteriorating upper renal tracts and renal function due to congenital or neuropathic abnormalities of the lower urinary tract. The former group may offer a later challenging problem should undiversion be considered.

In the older age group, urinary diversion combined with radiotherapy and cystourethrectomy may be attempting cure of malignant disease or may be a salvage procedure to relieve intolerable lower urinary tract symptoms caused by either the disease or its treatment.

Urologists may very reasonably adopt one of two alternative attitudes to urinary diversion. The first is to confine one's surgery to a single technique, most commonly a free draining ileal conduit with an urostomy appliance. The rationale is that over many years this will give increasing experience and technical expertise to ensure good and reliable results with a minimum of morbidity or mortality. Attention to detail is undeniably important with any form of urinary diversion. It is appropriate that recognition should be given to Eugene Bricker for his pioneer work in developing the ileal conduit and to his excellent recent review article (Bricker 1980) of his personal experience with ileal conduits during the last 30 years. This illustrates very clearly how small changes in the details of his own technique have produced increasingly good results.

It is true that there are few occasions when an ileal conduit is not technically possible, or indeed a perfectly acceptable form of urinary diversion, but there is a place for a second approach to urinary diversion, in which the urologist contemplates and selects what is judged to be the best technique available for an individual patient.

Bricker EM (1980) Current status of urinary diversion. Cancer 45: 2986–2991

This attitude is favoured by the contributors to this volume.

It is very pertinent that David Thomas and Tony Rickwood in their chapter on Neuro-Vesical Dysfunction, present data which should encourage urologists to rethink their approach to the timing of urinary diversion in cases with neuropathic bladders, particularly in children. It is just as important in this volume, to emphasise a swing towards a conservative non-operative management as it is to discuss advances in operations and surgical technique. Evidence is presented to favour a trial of intermittent self-catheterisation of the retaining neuropathic bladder, to avoid overflow incontinence and protect the upper renal tracts from reflux, backpressure hydronephrosis, pyelonephritis and deterioration of renal function.

Comparable to the wide choice of urinary diversions available to the surgeon, Thomas emphasises that 'a conservative regime must be based on a sound understanding of pathophysiological principles and that each patient must be considered individually and not slotted onto some preconceived classification of neurovesical dysfunction'. It will do no surgeon any harm to be told to 'learn the pharmacological skills of the physician'.

Thomas and Rickwood conclude from their personal experience in the Spinal Injuries Unit in Sheffield, that urinary diversion should only be considered if there is a failure of both intermittent self-catheterisation and pharmacological drugs to control detrusor and urethral sphincter dysfunction. Urinary diversion in children is therefore considered only as a last resort to try to preserve renal function.

The disappointing long-term results for both ileal and colonic urinary conduits in children are now well known and are confirmed by Rickwood's survey of the Sheffield results. Attention to detail of both operative technique and long-term postoperative management are important. The choice between a reflux preventing or refluxing ureteroileal anastomosis remains one of personal preference, whilst a non-refluxing ureterocolic anastomosis is favoured by most urologists. It is more important to avoid ureteric stenosis and a variety of techniques for uretero-bowel anatomoses are discussed.

With advances in both reconstructive urology and urodynamic assessment of a defunctioned bladder *undiversion* will become increasingly important. A large number of ingenious reconstructive procedures have been described but they may prove ill-judged unless preoperative assessment has shown a well motivated patient with a bladder of adequate capacity and good sphincter control.

Both Tony Walsh and I, in our respective chapters, emphasise that the choice of urinary diversion may vary with the socio-economic and environmental differences in the Western as opposed to Eastern or Third World countries. What is acceptable to one may be totally unacceptable to another and may include a complete rejection of any wet cutaneous stoma. This justifies attempts to develop a reliable, appliance free, urinary diversion, ranging from the often maligned ureterosigmoidostomy to one of the more experimental urinary reservoirs emptied by intermittent self catheterisation via a continent cutaneous stoma. The alternative choice between a free-draining urinary conduit or a colostomy and rectal bladder remains one of personal preference between the patient and surgeon and Walsh refers in detail to the work of Ghoneim in Egypt on this problem in a country where bilharzia is rife.

Whilst agreeing that in many cases, a one-stage cystourethrectomy and urinary diversion can be done, Walsh discusses his considerable personal experience with staged urinary diversion in the elderly unfit patient. It may be that future developments in oncology will alter our criteria for total cystectomy and allow an increase in numbers of partial cystectomies or subtotal cystectomies and cystoplasties to maintain continent micturition per urethram.

Experimental work using artificial scaffolds for bladder regeneration have so far not achieved clinical support and the insertion of subcutaneous magnets to produce a continent stoma is still in the experimental stage. Similarly, work in California and Tübingen with urinary conduits utilising pure vitreous carbon have been encouraging with vesicostomies in dogs, and clinical trials are underway in humans, but the long term problems of encrustation may persist. Biocarbon is theoretically inert to urine and well tolerated by urothelium, and the spout can be attached to an urostomy appliance without any risk of stenosis or the need for skin adhesives or belts.

The emergence of clinical nurses specialising in stoma care is a major advance in the management of patients undergoing urinary diversions. With tactful co-operation, it is made possible for the stomatherapist to visit patients in the ward both pre- and post-operatively, to discuss, demonstrate and select the most appropriate urostomy appliance for that particular patient. The design and materials of these appliances are continually improving. It is essential that the stomatherapist has a co-operative access to these patients both in the hospital and at the patient's home. This approach is expanded by Auriol Lawson and endorsed by Tony Walsh, with the plea that every Urological Unit should have the establishment for a stoma nurse in their area. We should be sceptical of the surgeon 'whose stomas never give any trouble' and who merely asks the patient in a busy out-patient clinic 'if all is well' without examining the stoma often hidden by the urostomy bag. Our patients are often our most loyal supporters and may be reluctant to complain about minor but still important practical stoma problems, for fear of 'letting their surgeon down'!

Each chapter in this volume represents the results and thoughts of considerable personal experience. This is exemplified by Michael Marberger and Eberhard Straub in their long-term review of ureterosigmoidostomy done in children in Mainz, with new data on both the growth development and psychological impact of ureterosigmoidostomy on these children.

Urinary diversion is not a subject for dogmatic or didactic teaching. It requires a wide ranging appraisal both of non-operative conservative management and of aggressive surgical procedures, in dealing with a major world-wide urological problem. We have tried to avoid repetition unless points are considered worthy of especial emphasis.

I was trained and stimulated in my urological thought by Richard Turner-Warwick. He always emphasised that technical expertise alone is not enough, but equally important is knowing which operation to advise for an individual patient. We hope this volume will encourage and stimulate this approach to urinary diversion.

Acknowledgements

I would like to express my sincere thanks to all the contributors of this volume, both for the personal expertise of their chapters and for their readiness to co-operate throughout this project. We all wish to record our appreciation to our respective secretaries for their patience and good humour in the typing and retyping of the texts and to our Departments of Photography and Medical Illustration for their willing help, especially mentioning Mr. Patrick M. Elliott, Senior Medical Artist at the Royal Hallamshire Hospital, Sheffield, whose illustrations appear throughout this volume.

Michael Jackson from Springer-Verlag and Geoffrey Chisholm in Edinburgh have been a constant source of encouragement, helping to maintain the enthusiasm of the contributors and giving experienced guidance to the editor. Finally, we are all indebted to our wives and children for forebearance in yet another Urological project to dilute the precious and all too short time available for us to spend with our families.

Norwich, January 1982   Michael Handley Ashken

Contents

Contributors

Michael Handley Ashken, BSc, MS, FRCS
Consultant Urologist, Norfolk and Norwich Hospital, Norwich,
Norfolk, England.

Auriol L. Lawson, SRN, JBCHS
Clinical Nurse Specialist in Stoma Care, Freeman Hospital,
Newcastle-upon-Tyne, England.

Michael Marberger, MD
Chief, Department of Urology, Krankenanstalt Rudolfstiftung;
Consultant-Urologist, Preyer'sches Children's Hospital, Vienna,
Austria.

Anthony M. K. Rickwood, MA, FRCS
Consultant Surgeon, Spinal Injuries Unit, Lodge Moor Hospital,
Sheffield, England.

Eberhard Straub, MD
Professor, Department of Pediatrics, University of Mainz Medical
School, Mainz, Germany.

David G. Thomas, MB, BS, FRCS
Consultant Urologist, Lodge Moor Hospital, Sheffield, England.

Anthony Walsh, FRCSI
Consultant Urologist, Jervis Street Hospital, Dublin, Eire.

Chapter 1

Urinary Diversion and Neuro-Vesical Dysfunction

David G. Thomas and Anthony M. K. Rickwood

Introduction

The most frequent reason for performing conduit urinary diversion has been, and remains, cystectomy for malignant disease. Probably the commonest reason for urinary diversion in non-malignant disease has been incontinence or upper tract deterioration related to neuro-vesical dysfunction. The choice of past tense is deliberate in this context where urinary diversion, always more widely used in treating patients with congenital rather than acquired lesions of the cord, is now viewed with increasing disfavour (Smith 1972; Zachary and Lister 1972; Guttman 1974). This reluctance to perform conduit diversion has been motivated largely by the development of alternative methods of treatment, but the emerging, and often disturbing, results of long-term follow up of conduit-diverted patients has added considerable support to the conservative approach (Middleton and Hendren 1976; Dunn et al. 1979; Elder et al. 1979; Pitts and Muecke 1979). The past decade has seen an increasing interest in the pathophysiology of neuro-vesical dysfunction mainly as a consequence of modern urodynamic investigation but also a renewed interest in the pharmacological manipulation of vesical and urethral function. The surgeon has come to learn that the pharmacological skills of the physician often have surprising and gratifying results.

In any centre with more than just a passing interest in neurological urology, urinary conduit diversion can now be regarded as a failure of conservative management, particularly in patients with non-progressive neurological disease. There are, naturally, exceptions to this generalisation and these will be discussed in this chapter.

In parallel with a growing disenchantment with permanent urinary diversion there has been an appreciation that a proportion of patients so treated in the past, including some with neuro-vesical dysfunction, retain a bladder capable of useful function and there are increasing reports of 'undiversion' in such cases.

Whilst it is not intended to provide a comprehensive guide to the management of patients with neuro-vesical dysfunction with such introductory remarks, some explanation and justification for a generally conservative approach must be provided, and it is hoped that this will help define the rather limited role that urinary diversion is now seen to play.

Causes of Neuro-Vesical Dysfunction

Although there are many features of neuro-vesical dysfunction common to all the various causes it is convenient to define the three general categories of neurological disease.

Congenital Cord Lesions

Myelomeningocoele
Lipoma of the Cauda Equina
Sacral agenesis
Diastematomyelia

Acquired Cord Lesions with Non-Progressive Neurological Deficit

Traumatic paraplegia and tetraplegia
Spinal artery thrombosis
Transverse Myelitis

Acquired Cord Lesions with Progressive Neurological Deficit

Multiple Sclerosis
Spinal cord tumours

Pathophysiology of Neuro-Vesical Dysfunction

The three main clinical features of neuro-vesical dysfunction, incontinence, failure of bladder emptying and upper renal tract complications, are all related to altered detrusor and sphincter function, and frequently co-exist.

Incontinence

Urethral leakage of urine in patients with neurological disease is almost always related to a combination of detrusor and urethral dysfunction but it is convenient to consider the two components separately.

Uninhibited detrusor contractions (Detrusor instability)

This is seen in patients with cord lesions which leave the sacral segments intact but totally or partially isolated (often associated with detrusor-sphincter dyssynergia) or with lesions higher in the neuraxis (usually with co-ordinated relaxation of the distal urethral sphincter). Uninhibited detrusor contractions may occur at any stage during filling but more often only at bladder capacity.

Sphincter Weakness Incontinence

This characteristically occurs with lesions destroying the sacral cord or cauda equina producing an acontractile detrusor with a flaccid paralysis of the pelvic floor muscles including the striated component of the distal urethral sphincter. Such incontinence may be made worse over a period of time by continued voiding by manual compression or abdominal straining.

Urethral Relaxation (Urethral Instability)

This is largely confined to female patients with multiple sclerosis in whom there is leakage of urine with no detectable rise in detrusor or intra-abdominal pressure.

Overflow Incontinence

Bladder neck and urethral incompetence in association with an overfull and usually acontractile bladder.

Failure in Bladder Emptying

Detrusor Acontractility

This occurs when a patient with an acontractile bladder fails to void by compression or straining.

Unsustained Detrusor Contractions

Detrusor contractions, whether occurring voluntarily or 'reflexly' may be poorly sustained and contribute towards poor bladder emptying.

Detrusor-Sphincter Dyssynergia

Failure of co-ordinated relaxation, or active contraction, of the striated component of the distal urethral sphincter during a detrusor contraction leads to functional urethral obstruction. This phenomenon may also include the pelvic floor and bulbar muscles and by definition occurs exclusively in patients with contractile bladders.

Distal Urethral Sphincter Obstruction

This is quite different from detrusor-sphincter dyssynergia. Although situated at the same anatomical level in the urethra it is associated with acontractile bladder and flaccid paralysis of all components of the striated musculature of the pelvic floor. Voiding by straining or compression is accompanied by failure of 'relaxation' of a relatively short segment of the distal urethral sphincter. The urethral component responsible for this obstruction would appear to have an alpha-adrenergic innervation and the outlet resistance may be reduced by alpha-adrenergic blockade (Awad et al. 1978).

Urethral Distortion

This situation is seen in patients with acontractile bladders where attempts to void by straining or compression result in acute obstructive kinking of the proximal urethra associated with the descent of the bladder base and pelvic floor.

Upper Renal Tract Dilatation (with or without Vesico-Ureteric Reflux)

High Residual Urine

Incomplete bladder emptying due to the variety of factors already mentioned may lead to upper tract deterioration.

Detrusor-Sphincter Dyssynergia

Although commonly accompanied by a high residual urine, upper tract dilatation may occur in the absence of any residual, especially when detrusor voiding pressures are high. This is seen most commonly in adult male patients with supra-sacral spinal cord lesions in the absence of vesico-ureteric reflux.

The 'Thick Walled' Bladder

Occasionally gross upper tract dilatation, without reflux, is seen with thick-walled acontractile bladders in the absence of a high residual urine. The bladder wall is usually non-compliant in the sense that there is a steady intravesical pressure rise during filling.

The Cord Lesion

For reasons which are not well understood dilatation of the upper renal tracts is uncommon in patients with progressive neurological disease, regardless of sex or the nature of the neuro-vesical dysfunction. Upper tract deterioration is most frequently encountered with patients with congenital cord lesions and almost invariably in association with a high residual urine. Vesico-ureteric reflux is particularly common in this group. Upper tract dilatation is less common following acquired cord lesions with non-progressive neurology, but is seen, not only in association with a high residual urine, but also with detrusor-sphincter dyssynergia with good bladder emptying.

Upper tract dilatation very rarely follows acquired cord lesions in female patients whereas in patients with congenital cord lesions both sexes seem almost equally at risk (Thomas and Clarke 1979).

Assessment of Neuro-Vesical Dysfunction

General Considerations

Any conservative regime of management should be based on a sound understanding of the pathophysiology of neuro-vesical dysfunction. Each patient must be considered individually and not slotted into some preconceived classification of neuro-vesical dysfunction. A careful history and accurate assessment of the neurological deficit is essential and must be complemented by objective assessment of detrusor and sphincter dysfunction, demonstrated by urodynamic and radiological studies.

Urodynamic Investigation

Most of the urodynamic investigations performed at the present time are directed towards problems of non-neurogenic female incontinence and male outflow tract obstruction. This involves the use of rapid single fill cystometry designed to detect detrusor instability. The techniques are quite inappropriate to the study of neuro-vesical dysfunction, which requires a less provocative and more physiological approach.

Residual Urine

In a patient with uninhibited detrusor activity (supra-sacral neurological lesions) with incomplete bladder emptying, drainage of residual urine prior to urodynamic study may radically alter the pattern of both 'reflex detrusor contractions' and detrusor-sphincter dyssynergia. The bladder should be filled on top of any existing residual urine.

Speed of Filling

The bladder with uninhibited detrusor activity often responds to rapid filling in an exaggerated fashion, with prolonged detrusor contractions occurring at an early stage of filling. This is usually quite unrepresentative of that bladder's normal performance at a physiological rate of filling.

Repeated Voiding Sequences

After insertion of a urethral catheter the first, and even the second, voiding sequence may be unrepresentative of the bladder's normal pattern of behaviour. It is advisable to use two fine (1.0–1.5 mm) catheters, one for filling and one for pressure measurement in order to be able to record a series of voiding sequences.

Radiological Studies

Combined urodynamic studies with synchronous imaging of the bladder and urethra provides a great deal of useful extra information on different aspects of detrusor and sphincter function.

Other Investigations

Measurement of urethral pressure profile or more specialised techniques such as detrusor or sphincter electromyography may produce additional information but are not part of our routine investigation of the neurogenic bladder.

Conservative Management of Neuro-Vesical Dysfunction

General Principles

It is essential to realise that the management of a neurogenic bladder cannot be divorced from consideration of the patient's overall neurological disabilities (mobility, use of hands, intelligence) and social circumstances and that any of these may themselves materially influence treatment. Management may also be determined by the nature of the neurological disease and the sex of the patient as they affect the likely risk to the upper renal tracts (B, III, 4). The sex of the patient also profoundly influences the attitude to incontinence, which, in general terms, can be managed in most adult males and older boys with a penile appliance, whereas no such facility exists for females.

The fundamental objectives of management are a continent patient with normal upper tracts. The latter must always take precedence, and in general terms is secured by measures designed to promote bladder emptying.

Measures to Promote Bladder Emptying

In patients with neurological disease the existence of a high residual urine is not necessarily an indication for treatment, but action is advisable when it constitutes a risk to the upper renal tract, causes urinary infections with constitutional upset, or is itself a major factor contributing to incontinence. It is also important to realise that dangerous outlet obstruction can occur in the absence of a high residual urine.

Drug Therapy

a) To improve detrusor activity (acontractile bladders, unsustained detrusor contractions).
Cholinergic agents such as carbachol and long acting anticholinesterase drugs such as distigmine bromide (Ubretid) may be useful as short or long-term therapy.

b) Reduction of outlet resistance (acontractile bladders). Alpha-adrenergic blockade may prove a most effective measure in reducing residual urine and upper tract dilatation (Fig. 1.1a,b). As a rule it is more likely to succeed in females and in young patients. The agent most commonly employed is phenoxybenzamine (Applebaum 1980).

Bladder Neck and Urethral Surgery

The usual site of outlet obstruction is at the level of the distal urethral sphincter and this is amenable to surgical treatment regardless of whether the bladder is contractile

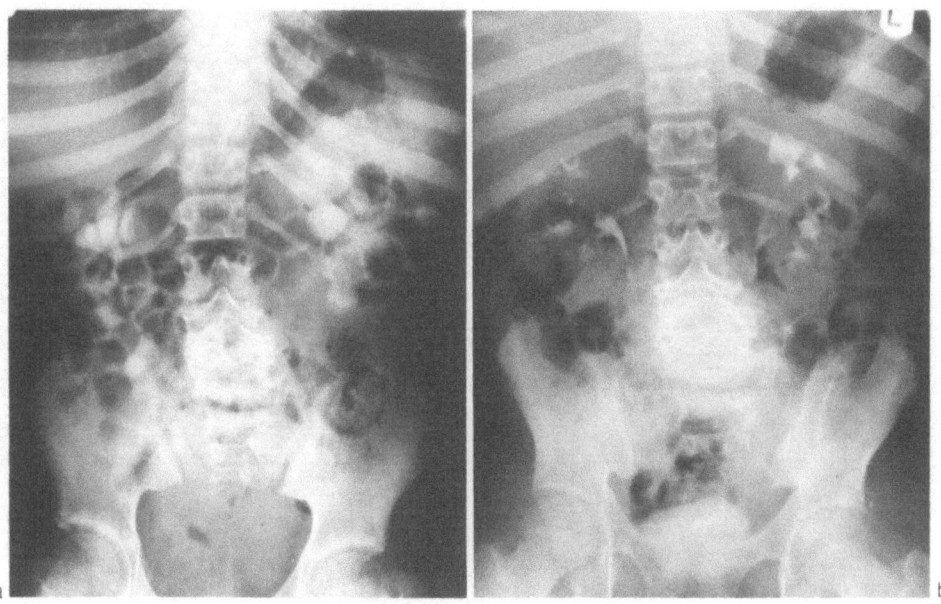

Fig.1.1 **a** Female aged 12 years, partial sacral agenesis plus diastematomyelia. Acontractile bladder, strains to void, residual urine 200 ml, incontinent. I.V.P. shows marked bilateral hydronephrosis. **b** I.V.P. after 1 year's treatment with phenoxybenzamine showing complete resolution of hydronephrosis. Residual urine zero, continent.

or acontractile. Bladder neck obstruction is rare; in the older male patient prostatic enlargement may occasionally prove an additional obstructive factor.

a) Endoscopic division of the distal urethral sphincter.
Division of the distal sphincter is now a well established means of reducing functional obstruction at this level, and is best performed using the resectoscope with an electrode knife. Antero-median incision (12 o'clock) is preferred to the 3 and 9 o'clock incisions, being much less likely to lead to post-operative erectile impotence. Gross upper tract dilatation in the presence (Fig. 1.2a–c) or absence (Fig. 1.3a–c) of vesico-ureteric reflux can be completely reversed by adequate sphincterotomy, and show lasting improvement.

b) Internal urethrotomy (Otis) and urethral dilatation (Rickwood 1981; Johnston and Kathel 1971).
In infants the upper renal tracts may show dramatic and lasting improvement following vigorous application of either of these techniques (Fig. 1.4a–c). They have no place in the treatment of older children or adults with neuro-vesical dysfunction.

Indwelling Urethral Catheters

(See p. 12).

Intermittent Catheterisation

(See p. 12).

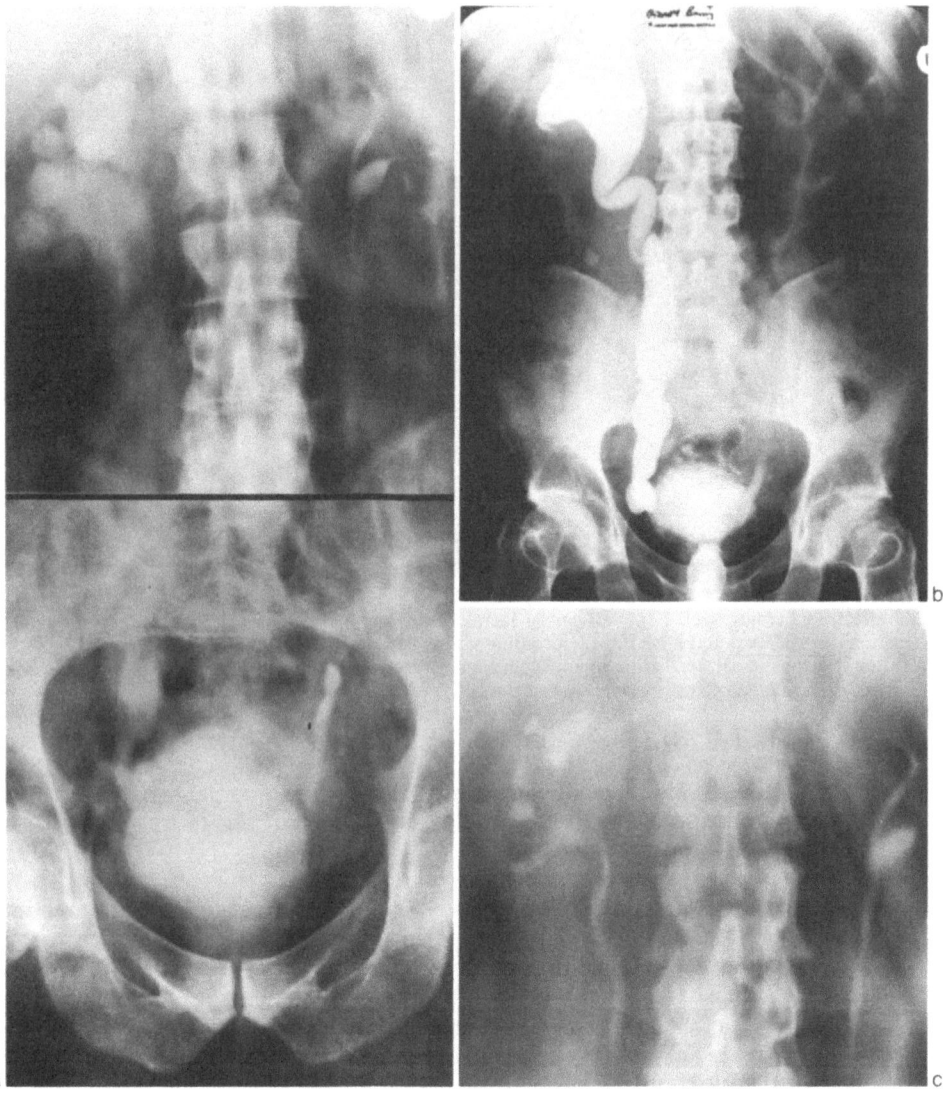

Fig.1.2. a Male paraplegic reflex micturition. I.V.P. showing right upper tract dilatation. **b** Same patient, cystogram; showing gross vesico-ureteric reflux plus detrusor sphincter dyssynergia. **c** Same patient. Post-sphincterotomy. I.V.P. showing considerable improvement in upper tract drainage but showing parenchymal damage.

Measures to Achieve Continence — General Principles

It is convenient to consider incontinence in relation to bladder capacity and the ability of the patient to void at will, either by voluntary detrusor control or 'reflex' detrusor contractions or straining/compression. Bladder sensation is not essential to full control but obviously extremely useful.

Methods Aimed at Improving Bladder Capacity — either by Reducing Detrusor Activity or by Increasing Urethral Activity

a) Drug therapy

Antispasmodic drugs — propantheline (Probanthine), emepronium bromide (Cetiprin), imipramine (Tofranil), flavoxate (Urispas), oxybutinin (Ditropan).

It may be necessary to use these drugs in large dosage, or in combination, in order to gain adequate suppression of detrusor activity. In our hands, imipramine has proved the most effective agent commercially available in the United Kingdom and this may be due, in part, to its secondary effect of increasing proximal urethral resistance (Mahoney et al. 1974; Khanna et al. 1975).

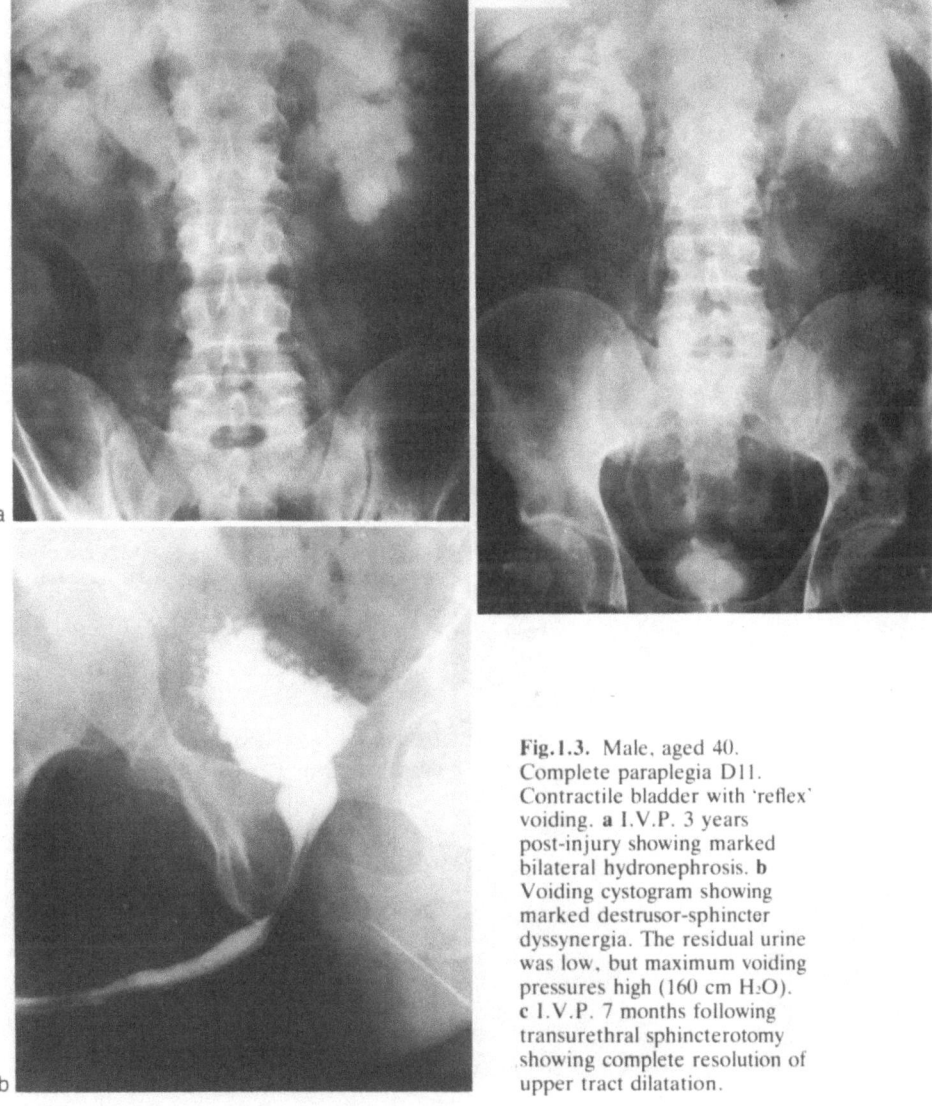

Fig.1.3. Male, aged 40. Complete paraplegia D11. Contractile bladder with 'reflex' voiding. **a** I.V.P. 3 years post-injury showing marked bilateral hydronephrosis. **b** Voiding cystogram showing marked destrusor-sphincter dyssynergia. The residual urine was low, but maximum voiding pressures high (160 cm H₂O). **c** I.V.P. 7 months following transurethral sphincterotomy showing complete resolution of upper tract dilatation.

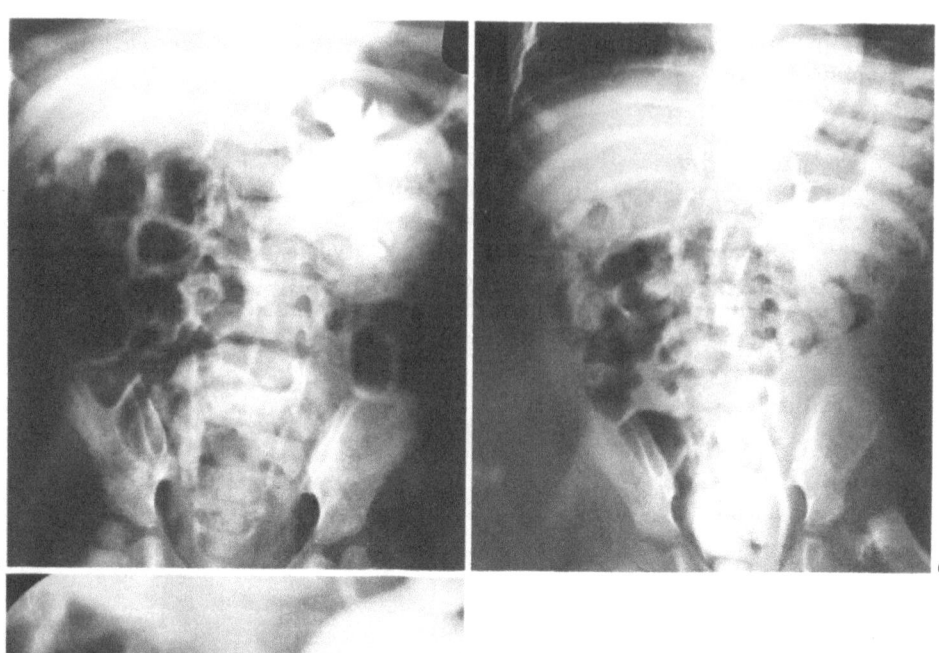

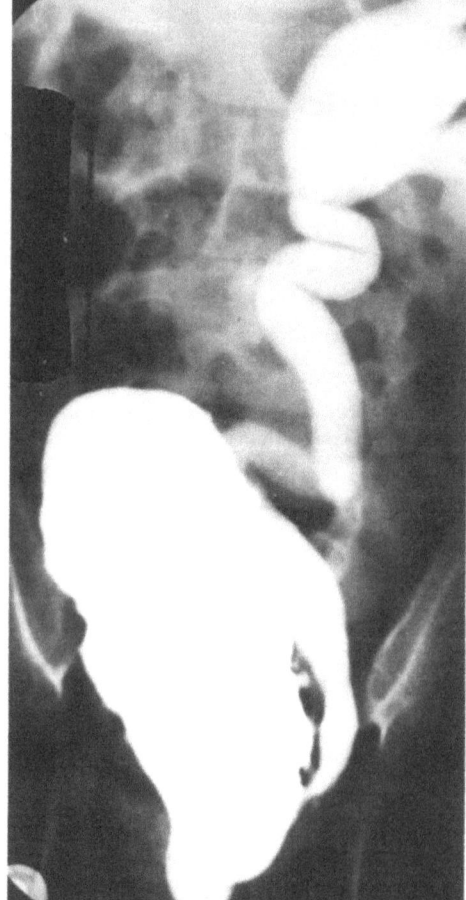

Fig. 1.4. a Female aged 2½
years, thoraco-lumbar myelomeningocoele, contractile
bladder, I.V.P. shows marked
hydronephrosis in solitary left
kidney. b Cystogram showing
severe vesico-ureteric reflux.
c I.V.P. 2 months after internal
(Otis) urethrotomy showing
almost complete resolution of
hydronephrosis. Four years
later the appearances are
maintained and a cystogram has
shown resolution of the
vesico-ureteric reflux.

Alpha-adrenergic blocking agents (ephedrine, phenylopropanolamine) are only of value when the major component producing incontinence is genuine sphincter weakness leakage. This is particularly the case in female patients with acontractile bladders or in females with urethral 'relaxation' as seen in multiple sclerosis.

Occasionally the paradoxical situation occurs when incontinence can be helped by the administration of drugs to increase detrusor activity and improve emptying. This is particularly so in the cases of incontinence related to large capacity, large residual bladders when improved emptying may abolish incontinence.

b) Ablative denervation procedures

i) Chemical Blocks

These may take the form of intra-thecal phenol or alcohol blocks, or more selective sacral root blockade, the choice being dependent on the degree of the existing neurological deficit.

ii) Surgical Denervation

Complete or selective sacral root section or peripheral denervation procedures often reduce detrusor overactivity and improve bladder capacity (Ingelman-Sundberg 1959; Torrens and Griffiths 1974; Clarke et al. 1979).

c) Bladder overdistension (Dunn et al. 1974: Ramsden et al. 1976).

Most of the reported results of this treatment relate to patients with detrusor instability in the absence of gross neurological disease. Its role in the treatment of neurological patients is yet to be evaluated.

d) Artificial sphincter

The first inflatable artificial sphincter was implanted in 1972 (Scott et al. 1973) and since that time the improved technical design has led to its increased usage in the United States. Careful patient selection is essential. When potential mechanical or infective problems are eliminated this type of treatment should be available for the correctly selected patient. The prosthesis can be used in male and female patients and does not interfere with male or female sexual function (Scott 1978; Furlow 1980).

Means of Voiding at Will

Voluntary Detrusor Contractions

A few patients with an incomplete neurological lesion retain this facility. In patients with congenital cord lesions this may not become apparent until the age of five years or later.

Abdominal Straining or Compression (Acontractile Bladders)

Straining to empty the bladder is only possible when there is good voluntary contraction of the abdominal muscles (motor level D.12 or lower). With higher neurological lesions, manual compression is required and many patients are incapable of managing this effectively. This makes them reliant on other people, a limiting factor if they are otherwise independent.

Triggering of 'Reflex' Detrusor Contractions

This is usually achieved with supra-pubic tapping but sometimes can only be achieved by perianal stimulation, and in females may be reinforced by abdominal compression or straining. Some adult patients with marked detrusor-sphincter dyssynergia find that they can relax the distal urethral sphincter spasm by inserting a finger into the anal canal or sometimes by supra-pubic tapping during a bladder contraction. For unknown reasons all these manoeuvres are usually quite ineffective in patients with congenital cord lesions. Both of these methods come within the general category of 'bladder training' an often sadly neglected means of improving the micturition difficulties of the neurologically disabled patient. For such satis-factory training it is necessary to have a well motivated and reasonably mobile patient.

Intermittent Self-Catheterisation (Lapides et al. 1971)

This very simple concept has, perhaps, been one of the major advances in treating patients with neuro-vesical dysfunction in the last decade. In our hands it is more satisfactory as a means for treating incontinence than upper tract dilatation. The technique requires proper tuition, initial enthusiastic support from medical and nursing staff, and a well-motivated patient with circumstances suitable for the performance of the technique.

Drug therapy to improve bladder capacity may be necessary to enable the successful use of intermittent self-catheterisation. Similarly, surgical procedures such as bladder denervation or colposuspension may render self catheterisation possible.

Electrical Bladder Stimulation

Although this technique of managing the problems of bladder emptying and incontinence is in its relative infancy, it offers exciting prospects for the treatment of selected patients with neuro-vesical dysfunction. The procedure of choice would appear to be sacral anterior root stimulation and already a small series of traumatic paraplegic patients have achieved continence with satisfactory bladder emptying by this method (Brindley 1980).

Measures to Promote Continence — Indwelling Urethral Catheter and Penile Appliance

The measures outlined in the previous sections, either used alone or in combination, are frequently successful in securing continence but it is to be admitted that this is not always so. Failures most commonly occur amongst tetraplegics, male patients with sphincter weakness incontinence, and male traumatic paraplegics with contractile bladders who generally lack the necessary motivation to become dry.

Permanent Indwelling Urethral Catheterisation

There is little doubt that the judicious and proper use of a permanent indwelling Foley catheter in the incontinent and disabled neurological patient can prove an

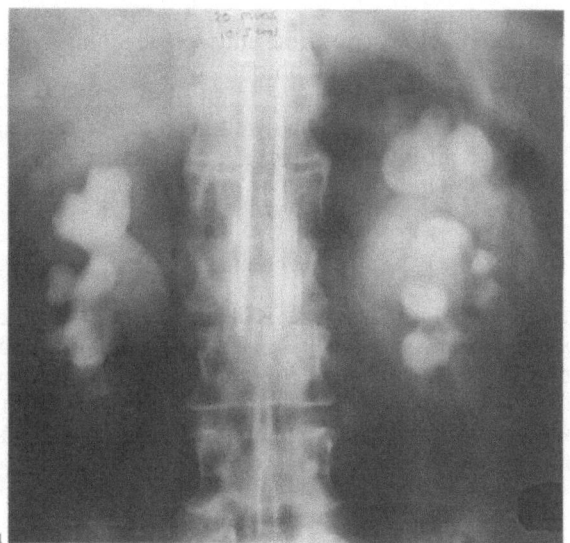

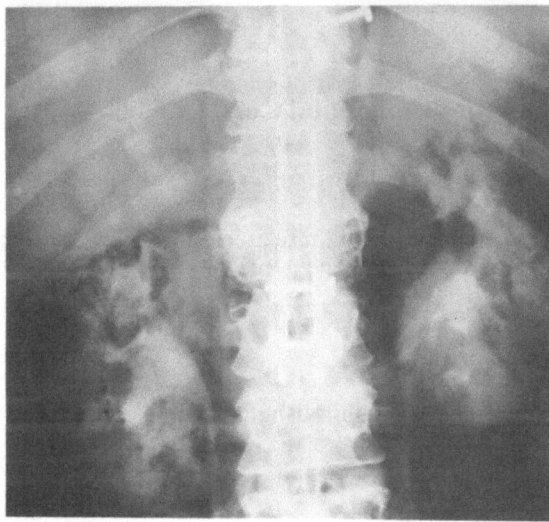

Fig.1.5. a Male, age 35, traumatic paraplegia, neurological level D.12 complete. Acontractile bladder with large residual urine. I.V.P. five years post-injury shows marked bilateral hydronephrosis. b A further I.V.P., 2 months after insertion of an indwelling catheter shows complete resolution of the hydronephrosis.

absolute blessing. The permanent catheter may have been provided primarily as a means of improving bladder emptying and hence the condition of the upper renal tracts (Fig. 1.5a,b), or purely as a means of achieving continence.

The complications which may arise are

a) Blockage due to stone or debris formation
b) Leakage around the catheter due to uninhibited detrusor contractions
c) Leakage due to a wide patulous urethra and bladder neck.

This last complication is usually avoidable and occurs as a result of the insertion of ever increasing catheter size and balloon size in futile attempts to overcome problems of leakage. In a bladder with uninhibited detrusor contractions the insertion of larger and larger catheters with larger balloon sizes often increases the detrusor irritability and increases the leakage.

In patients with permanent catheters cystoscopy and endoscopic stone removal may be necessary from time to time. Patients with uninhibited detrusor contractions producing problems often respond well to drug therapy and measures that have already been mentioned. Using these principles an indwelling catheter of appropriate size (for adults 18 F.G. with 5-ml balloon) proves a satisfactory means of securing continence for many years if not indefinitely.

Suprapubic Catheterisation

The use of permanent suprapubic bladder drainage is itself a form of urinary diversion but in a selected group of patients may be preferable to conduit diversion.

In female patients with uninhibited detrusor contractions producing incontinence despite continuous suprapubic catheter drainage it may be necessary to suture the bladder neck or urethra. An alternative manoeuvre avoiding urethral closure is the endoscopic elevation of the bladder neck (Stamey 1980).

Problems Peculiar to Patients with Congenital Cord Lesions

Certain features have already been mentioned but there are additional factors in this group of patients which can materially affect management.

Bladder Function

Whereas contractile bladders dominate in acquired neurological conditions, the reverse is true in congenital lesions.

Sex

Females predominate, marginally in myelomeningocoele, and markedly in lipoma of the cauda equina.

Age

Of necessity these patients require management from infancy to adult life. What may be adequate treatment for an infant (nappies) may be quite unsuitable for an older child or adult. With infants and young children management devolves largely on the parents, but, hopefully, self-management may be possible for older patients. The decisions as to management in children are apt to have very prolonged consequences, this is especially relevant with myelomeningocoele patients who survive following a selective policy of treatment, whose life expectancy is largely determined by the quality of management of the urinary tract.

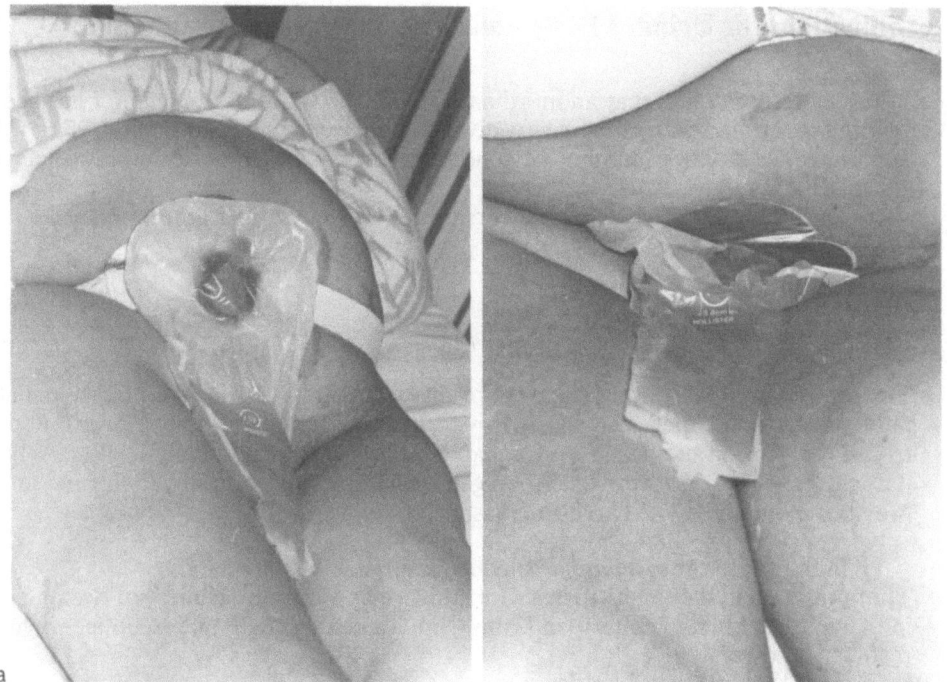

Fig.1.6. a Female aged 19 years. Thoracolumbar myelomeningocoele, wheelchair-bound. Ileal conduit performed at 2 years of age. There is a moderate lordo-scoliotic deformity and the stoma has been sited on the concave aspect of this. **b** When sitting the stoma retreats into the fold created by the spinal deformity and the appliance impinges on the thighs. The girl cannot fit her own appliances and is dependent on her parents, who find appliance management difficult, though not quite impossible. The stoma would have been better sited on the left and at a higher level.

Intelligence

Until the recent selective policy of treatment of neonates with myelomeningocoele was evolved (Lorner 1973), the great majority of surviving patients developed hydrocephalus requiring shunting procedures. As a group these patients are less intelligent than the population at large, lack initiative, and have poor manipulative skills. These factors must be borne in mind when considering treatment of bladder dysfunctions.

Spinal Deformity

The more extensive the original lesion the greater the chance of developing a spinal deformity. By their teens almost all patients with thoraco-lumbar lesions have developed a severe spinal deformity which may make the fitting of an appliance and an abdominal stoma a difficult or even impossible proposition (Fig. 1.6a,b).

Indications for Urinary Diversion in Neuro-Vesical Dysfunction

Some readers may feel that an inordinate amount of space in this chapter has been devoted to the alternatives to urinary diversion but we feel that subsequent years will see an ever decreasing number of conduit diversions being performed for neuro-vesical dysfunction.

The current reasons for urinary diversion can be summarised as follows:

Deterioration of the Upper Renal Tracts

This was formerly a common reason for diversion and the principal reason in male patients. In well supervised patients with neurovesical dysfunction, severe upper tract deterioration should rarely occur and is a largely avoidable complication. When it does happen, even severe examples generally respond favourably to the measures previously outlined. The two usual reasons for failure are:

1) Inability to secure adequate bladder emptying
There is usually a good reason for this (inappropriate choice of treatment, inadequate sphincterotomy) and this should be checked and rectified before resorting to diversion.

2) The 'thick-walled' bladder
Conservative management of upper tract dilatation in this situation is difficult if not impossible and diversion is often unavoidable.

Before undertaking diversion for upper tract dilatation it is always wise to ensure that this is due to obstruction rather than atony. Investigations such as isotope renography with diuresis (O'Reilly et al. 1978) and pressure/perfusion studies (Whitaker 1973) allow the two conditions to be distinguished with some degree of reliability. If the upper tracts prove to be atonic it is unlikely that diversion will be any more effective than continued conservative management.

Failure to Secure Continence

Male Patients

a) Small penis
It is exceedingly difficult, if not impossible, to use a penile appliance in small boys. Even older, active, boys may experience considerable problems. These difficulties should not themselves demand diversion; the long-term results of these procedures. are such that waiting until the patient is old enough to be satisfactorily fitted with an appliance is usually well worth while.

The problem of a small penis is relatively uncommon in adults but may produce some difficulties, particularly in older men with cervical cord injuries and young adult males with congenital cord lesions. In the latter the problem may be compounded by intractible obesity. For these few patients, provided there is no positive contraindication (e.g. severe spinal deformity) diversion may be preferred to an indwelling urethral catheter.

b) Anterior urethral fistula

Occasionally a badly fitting penile appliance may cause an anterior urethral fistula. Any surgical repair is liable to break down if a condom-type applicance is refitted to the penis and under these circumstances urinary diversion may be the best policy.

Female Patients

a) Patulous urethra and bladder neck

Although this complication is usually due to bad catheter management, and hence potentially avoidable, this problem continues to occur. Once established only a suprapubic catheter with urethral closure or permanent conduit diversion will solve the problem.

b) Other catheter problems

Despite every endeavour a few patients continue to experience intractible problems with catheter drainage (blockage or leakage) and under such circumstances conduit diversion is necessary to improve the quality of life.

Problems Related to Particular Neurological Conditions

Female Patients with Progressive Neurological Disease

In these patients, who often have a limited life expectancy, early diversion may be indicated when simple conservative measures have failed (Desmond and Shuttleworth 1977). It should be remembered that many of these patients have lost, or will lose, the use of their hands, and before undertaking diversion, firm assurance from relatives for continuing stoma care must be obtained.

Male Patients with Non-Progressive Neurological Disease

In a small number of male patients with good recovery of a cord lesion there is progressive upper tract dilatation but good preservation of sexual function. In such cases endoscopic division of the distal urethral sphincter may possibly impair sexual function although the risk is much smaller with the antero-median sphincterotomy. In such cases due consideration must be given to conduit diversion.

Patient Choice

It is unusual to find adults willing to accept major elective surgery without good reason. It is exceedingly rare for a male patient to request diversion but there are a few female patients who may find conduit diversion a more socially acceptable alternative to conservative management. They are usually the females who are managed without a catheter but find the discipline and effort to empty their bladders regularly and keep dry is more trouble than it is worth. Occasionally a female patient may regard an indwelling urethral catheter with more repugnance than an abdominal stoma. Faced with a request of this nature from the patient the surgeon can only discuss the pros and cons with the patients and their relatives as they apply in the particular case.

Types of Diversion Applicable in Neuro-Vesical Dysfunction

Vesical Diversions

As a means of handling upper tract dilatation vesical diversion would offer no material advantage over conservative measures, and is most unlikely to effect any improvement when the problem is due to a 'thick-walled' bladder.

As a means of treating incontinence a vesical diversion such as a suprapubic catheter is a comparatively minor procedure, especially applicable to the elderly and the frail. It may also be particularly suitable for patients with a severe spinal deformity. Regardless of the type of vesical diversion, if there is a severe degree of sphincter weakness incontinence or detrusor instability it may be necessary to obliterate the bladder outlet. In females this can be fairly reliably achieved by circumcising the external urethral meatus and mobilising the urethra sufficiently to be able to invaginate it with two layers of pursestring sutures. A similar technique has been described for males but mobilising the urethra downwards from the bladder neck (Reid et al. 1978). An alternative for females is endoscopic elevation of the bladder neck (Stamey 1980).

Cutaneous Ureterostomy

Once commonly used in patients with congenital cord lesions (Lister et al. 1968; Eckstein and Kapila 1970) this procedure is now almost obsolete. It is only applicable when at least one ureter is massively and chronically dilated, an event which should now be rare and in any case is usually reversible by conservative measures. Loop ureterostomy as a definitive means of dealing with unilateral dilatation is to be condemned; the effect on the upper tract may be satisfactory but the patient is left having to cope with an abdominal stoma and an incontinent bladder. Nearly all such procedures have subsequently required undiversion or conversion to some form of conduit diversion.

Cutaneous ureterostomy may still occasionally be indicated in children in the following circumstances:

1) When one or both upper tracts remain massively dilated (but not aperistaltic) following adequate conservative treatment. An end-ureterostomy in this situation is a comparatively minor procedure and the long term results appear to be no worse than those following conduit diversion. Should the occasion ever arise, they are usually relatively easy to undivert.

2) A loop, ring or Sober ureterostomy may be a useful temporising measure in boys with massive upper tract dilatation in association with neuro-vesical dysfunction of obscure origin (the so called 'Occult Neuropathic Bladder') when it is considered inadvisable to perform some irreversible procedure such as endoscopic sphincterotomy or permanent diversion.

Conduit Diversions

As long as urinary diversion plays any role in the management of neuro-vesical dysfunction, the conduit is likely to remain the most popular procedure, being applicable to most situations. In the past, the choice of conduit was largely dictated by choice of stoma site, but there are other considerations worth mentioning.

1) Ileal conduit

In adults this is generally considered a safer procedure than the colonic conduit. It is usually constructed in such a way as to allow free ureteric reflux. This may be of limited consequence in adults, especially where life expectancy is limited, but in children, the long term results of refluxing conduits are so poor that this procedure cannot be recommended except as a last resort.

2) Colonic conduits

Sigmoid colon is usually used, and it is true that in patients with long standing neurological disease this portion of the bowel becomes somewhat redundant and is technically easy to isolate as a conduit. It may be questioned, however, whether such chronically dilated colon will function satisfactorily as a conduit.

The advantage claimed for the colonic conduit is that it lends itself to reliable anti-refluxing uretero-intestinal anastomosis, and some medium term follow-up suggests that in children, non-refluxing conduits secure better preservation of renal function (Altwein et al. 1977; Althausen et al. 1978).

Continent Reservoirs

These have been employed only on a limited scale in patients with neurological disease, but may have a particular role to play in the patient who is unable to use a collecting appliance by virtue of a severe spinal deformity.

In a small number of patients who find urethral self-catheterisation difficult, a leak-proof vesicostomy has been constructed by Turner-Warwick (1976). An intra-vesical everted spout of ileum was created to act as a valve with a short length of ileum passing to a dry skin stoma. This was best placed on the posterior wall of the bladder to help an easy self-catheterisation and was very satisfactory in patients with large capacity acontractile bladders who could not manage urethral self-catheter-isation. A leak-proof vesicostomy proved disappointing for the management of unstable detrusor incontinence because the involuntary detrusor contractions became acutely painful when they could no longer create a urinary leakage.

Practical Considerations of Conduit Diversion in Neurological Disease

The technical aspects of the various type of diversion used in patients with neurological disease are covered elsewhere in this volume. Certain features relevant to patients with neurological disease are worth mentioning.

Bowel Preparation

Many patients become extremely constipated with a redundant sigmoid colon and clearance of the colon may be extremely difficult and prolonged. Time spent in good bowel preparation is always time well spent.

Siting the Stoma

In patients without spinal deformity this presents no particular problems. Special care is necessary in patients with congenital cord lesions in whom spinal deformities are common.

Age of Patient

In adolescents any deformity will be fully developed and the nature of the problem is immediately evident. This is not so in younger children, where the spine, on superficial inspection, may appear almost straight. It is essential to bear in mind that any deformity in a young child will certainly become worse by adolescence. How much so depends largely on the extent of the original spinal lesion and is likely to be particularly severe in the presence of hemi-vertebrae. In young children the direction of the deformity can be gauged from abdominal X-rays even when it is not evident clinically.

Lordosis

This proves the least difficult deformity from the point of view of appliance management. It is advisable to avoid a low stoma site, which, in the sitting position, will cause the appliance to impinge on the patient's thighs.

Kyphosis

It is vital not to site the stoma in the abdominal fold caused by the kyphos. If there is any choice the stoma is best sited above the fold.

Scoliosis

As a general rule the stoma should be sited on the convex side of a scoliotic deformity.

Compound Deformities

These call for considerable judgement, and in some cases defy all attempts at finding a satisfactory site.

Shunts for Hydrocephalus

In patients with shunted hydrocephalus the lower catheter is often placed intra-peritoneally, and presents when the abdomen is opened for a conduit. In the authors' experience provided it is tucked well away into the upper abdomen at the beginning of the procedure, there is no risk of an ascending shunt infection and no need to give prophylactic antibiotics.

References

Althausen AF, Hagenlook K, Hendren WH (1978) Non-refluxing colon conduit: Experience with 70 cases. J Urol 120: 35–39

Altwein JE, Jonas U, Hohenfellner R (1977) Long-term follow up of children with colon conduit urinary diversions and ureterosigmoidostomy. J Urol 118: 832–836

Applebaum SM (1980) Pharmacological agents in micturitional disorders. Urology 16: 555–568

Awad SA, Downie JW, Kiruluta HG (1978) Alpha-adrenergic agents in urinary disorders of the proximal urethra. 1. Sphincteric incontinence. Br J Urol 50: 332–335

Clarke SJ, Forster DMC, Thomas DG (1979) Selective sacral neurectomy in the management of urinary incontinence due to detrusor instability. Br J Urol 51: 510–514

Desmond AD, Shuttleworth KED (1977) The results of urinary diversion in multiple sclerosis. Br J Urol 49: 495–502

Dunn M, Smith JC, Ardran GM (1974) Prolonged bladder distension as a treatment of urgency and urge incontinence of urine. Br J Urol 46: 645–652

Dunn M, Roberts JBM, Smith PJB, Slade N (1979) The long term results of ileal conduit diversion in children. Br J Urol 51: 306–315

Eckstein HB, Kapila L (1970) Cutaneous ureterostomy. Br J Urol 42: 306–315

Elder DD, Moisey CU, Rees RWM (1979) A long term follow up of the colonic conduit operation in children. Br J Urol 51: 462–465

Furlow WL (1980) Artificial sphincter. In: Stanton SL, Tanagho EA (eds) Surgery of female incontinence. Springer, Berlin Heidelberg New York, pp 119–134

Guttmann L (1974) Spinal cord injuries. Blackwell Scientific, Oxford, pp 306–429

Ingelman-Sundberg A (1959) Partial denervation of the bladder. A new method for the treatment of urge incontinence and similar conditions in women. Acta Obstet Gynecol Scand 38: 487–502

Johnston JH, Kathel BL (1971) The obstructed neurogenic bladder in the new born. Br J Urol 43: 206–210

Khanna OP, Elkous G, Heber D, Gonick P (1975) Imipramine hydrochloride. Pharmacodynamic effects in lower urinary tract of female dogs. Urology 6: 48–52

Lapides J, Diokno AC, Silber SJ (1971) Clean, intermittent self-catheterization in the treatment of urinary tract disease. Trans Am Assoc Genitourin Surg 63: 92–95

Lister J, Cook RCM, Zachary RB (1968) Operative management of neurogenic bladder dysfunction in children: Ureterostomy. Arch Dis Child 43: 672–678

Lorber J (1973) Early results of selective treatment of spina bifida. Br Med J iv: 201–204

Mahoney DT, Laferte RO, Mahoney JE (1973) VI. Observations in sphincter-augmenting effect of imipramine in children with urinary incontinence. Urology 1: 317–323

Middleton AW, Hendren WH (1976) Ileal conduits in children at the Massachusetts General Hospital from 1955 to 1970. J Urol 115: 591–595

O'Reilly PH, Testa HJ, Lawson RS, Farrar DJ, Charlton-Edwards E (1978) Diuresis renography in equivocal urinary tract obstruction. Br J Urol 50: 76–80

Pitts WR Jr, Muecke EC (1979) A 20 year experience with ileal conduits — the fate of the kidneys. J Urol 122: 154–157

Ramsden PD, Smith JC, Dunn M, Ardran GM (1976) Distension therapy for the unstable bladder: Later results including an assessment of repeat distensions. Br J Urol 48: 623–629

Reid R, Schneider K, Fruchtman B (1978) Closure of the bladder neck in patients undergoing continent vesicostomy for urinary incontinence. J Urol 120: 40–42

Rickwood AMK (1981) Use of internal urethrotomy to reverse upper renal tract dilatation in children with neurogenic bladder dysfunction. Br J Urol awaiting publication

Scott FB (1978) The artificial sphincter in the management of incontinence in the male. Urol Clin North Am 5: 375–391

Scott FB, Bradley WE, Timm GW (1973) Treatment of urinary incontinence by implantable prosthetic sphincter. Urology 1: 252–259

Smith ED (1972) Follow up studies of 150 ileal conduits in children. J Pediatr Surg 7: 1–10

Stamey TA (1980) Endoscopic suspension of the vesical neck. In: Stanton SL, Tanagho EA (eds) Surgery of female incontinence. Springer, Berlin Heidelberg New York, pp. 77–91

Thomas DG, Clarke SJ (1979) The urological status of 86 females following spinal cord injury. Br J Urol 51: 515–517

Torrens MJ, Griffiths HB (1974) The control of the uninhibited bladder by selective sacral neurectomy. Br J Urol 46: 639–644

Turner-Warwick R (1976) Leak-proof cystostomy. J Urol Nephrol (Paris) 2 [Suppl 8]: 405–413

Whitaker RH (1973) Methods of assessing obstruction in dilated ureters. Br J Urol 45: 15–22

Zachary RB, Lister J (1972) Conservative management of the neurogenic bladder. In: Johnston JH Scholtmeijer RJ (eds) Problems in paediatric urology. Excerpta Medica, Amsterdam, pp 121–133

Chapter 2

Urinary Diversion in Children

Anthony M. K. Rickwood

Thirty years ago urinary diversion in a child was a rare event, virtually limited to ureterosigmoidostomy in a few patients with bladder extrophy. Two factors were soon to dramatically increase their number. Numerically more important was the advent of effective shunting devices for treating hydrocephalus, which, for more than a decade, were used widely, aggressively and often indiscriminately, to enable the survival of large numbers of patients with open spina bifida. One of many results of this policy was that the congenital neuropathic bladder, once rare, became commonplace. Faced with an epidemic of incontinent girls and an alarming number of children of both sexes with deteriorating upper renal tracts, it is small wonder that surgeons saw the ileal conduit (Bricker 1950) as an ideal solution to both problems (Nash 1956).

The second, and numerically less important factor, was the increasing interest in 'megaureters' from whatever cause and the realisation that these lent themselves to a miscellany of direct cutaneous diversions (Johnston 1963; Williams and Rabinovitch 1967; Eckstein and Kapila 1970). By 1970 a large number of children had undergone urinary diversion, temporary, or more commonly 'permanent', with results that were for the most part considered satisfactory (Kafetsioulis and Swinney 1968; Mogg and Syme 1969; Ray and de Dominico 1972; Smith 1972; Stevens and Eckstein 1977). The last decade has seen something of a reversal of these trends, with a growing appreciation that the long-term results of diversion in children are rather less than ideal (Scott 1973; Middleton and Hendren 1976; Hendren 1978b; Dunn et al. 1979; Elder et al. 1979; Pitts and Muecke 1979), an increased understanding of conditions for which diversion was previously advocated and a willingness to explore alternative methods of management.

General Considerations

The paramount concern must be that for a child a 'permanent' diversion should provide satisfactory drainage of the kidneys for a very long time, 60 years and more, if the procedure is purely for incontinence, and life expectancy is otherwise normal. Very few diversions so far performed approach even half this figure.

Children tolerate major surgery well, physically and psychologically. Common hazards in adult practice, chest infections, deep vein thrombosis, pulmonary embolism and vascular disease, are rare or absent. Technical problems are minimised by small amounts of fat, good vascularity of tissues and rapid healing. Given adequate supporting staff, a surgeon can be confident that the young patient will survive a major procedure, such as an ileal conduit, rapidly and with few complications. Admirable though this is, it serves as something of a temptation to indulge in radical surgery when a lesser procedure would suffice.

Surprisingly little attention has been given to the psychological aspects of diversion. The child appears to adapt remarkably quickly, but parents often less so, especially if there are practical problems or if they had not understood the nature of the procedure (Woodburn 1973). Smith (1965) advocates early diversion for incontinence on the grounds that whereas young patients grow up to accept an abdominal stoma, older children are disturbed by the idea. The policy in Sheffield has been to divert for incontinence only when it is clear to all concerned that this cannot be managed otherwise. In this way the benefits of diversion are more positively appreciated by parents and child and, usually, still well remembered by the patient as she passes through her teens. It is perhaps for this reason that we have largely avoided stoma rejection by teenagers (Dunn et al. 1979), although occasional examples have been seen in adolescents diverted in infancy for upper renal tract problems.

Almost inevitably, few children undergoing diversion for this indication can have any appreciation of its necessity, but it is important that the parents understand and the patient also, when old enough to do so.

Diversionary Procedures in Children

Most of the procedures described will be familiar to urologists and attention will be focussed on details of technique that are specific to children. The previous distinction between temporary and permanent diversions is no longer valid — most 'permanent' diversions are potentially reversible while not a few 'temporary' diversions remain permanent. The procedures will therefore be described in anatomical sequence.

Nephrostomy

Because of the infection which inevitably accompanies any form of intubated diversion, nephrostomy should only be considered as a last resort in the long and even medium term. Nevertheless it provides excellent drainage of the kidney, and as a short-term measure may be invaluable either to decompress a severely obstructed kidney prior to early definitive surgery or as a means of covering a reconstructive procedure on the upper urinary tract. Percutaneous techniques for inserting nephrostomy tubes under radiological or ultrasonic guidance have been described (Babcock et al. 1979; Sadlowski et al. 1979), but in the circumstances usually necessitating nephrostomy in a child, the more certain open procedure is preferred.

In children it is generally easier to approach the renal pelvis anteriorly especially when it is grossly dilated. With the patient tilted 30° toward the opposite side and a sandbag under the loin to open out the angle between ribs and pelvis, a short transverse muscle cutting incision is made from the lateral edge of the rectus sheath towards the tip of the 12th rib. Sweeping the peritoneum medially exposes the anterior renal pelvis which is opened between stay sutures, and a Malecot catheter is drawn in retrogradely through the lower polar calyx. A size 14F is satisfactory for babies and up to 18F in older children. No additional drainage is required.

Cutaneous Ureterostomy

This procedure may only be performed without risk of stenosis or ischaemic necrosis on ureters which are massively and chronically dilated — thick walled, vascular and tortuous. The acutely dilated ureter, thin walled, flabby and straight is no more suitable for cutaneous ureterostomy than one which is non- or minimally dilated (Johnston 1963).

Loop Ureterostomy

This is almost always intended as a temporary diversion. Siting is important: for the most severely affected upper tract a high ureterostomy in the flank provides the best hope of stabilising renal function (Johnston 1963) and does not usually interfere with any procedure that may later be required on the distal ureter prior to closure. Unfortunately it is difficult to manage stomal appliances at this site and for patients whose renal function proves too poor for undiversion, this may entail a rather tedious and hazardous conversion to an alternative type of diversion. In less severe circumstances, ureterostomy at a lower level provides adequate drainage and can be fashioned at a satisfactory stoma site but difficulties are encountered if later reimplantation of the ureter is required (Hendren 1978b). In this situation it is usually better to detach the ureter from the bladder and form an end ureterostomy with a view to subsequent direct reimplantation (Williams and Rabinovitch 1967).

The approach for high loop ureterostomy is similar to nephrostomy, except that the skin is incised obliquely downwards and medially and may incorporate a 'V' for a skin bridge (Fig. 2.1a). Proximally the ureter is straightened as far as the renal pelvis by dividing numerous filmy adhesions. Distal dissection need only be sufficient to enable the loop of the ureter to lie at skin level without tension. The muscle layers are lightly approximated and the skin bridge brought beneath the apex of the loop. A muscle bridge can be incorporated for additional security, but is unnecessary if ureteric mobilisation has been adequate and adds to the difficulties of subsequent closure. At the end of the procedure the apex of the loop is incised longtitudinally for some 2cm and the edges sutured to the skin (Fig. 2.1b). No internal drainage of the ureter is needed.

Sober (1972) and Ring Ureterostomies (Williams and Cromie 1975)

After total urinary diversion (including bilateral loop ureterostomies where only a little urine spills over into the distal limbs) the defunctioned bladder may become irreversibly contracted and require augmentation before undiversion can be considered (Lome et al. 1972). These procedures are intended to overcome this difficulty and to make for easier closure at a later stage. The approach and initial mobilisation of the ureter is as for loop ureterostomy. In the Sober procedure, the ureter is divided at a point where the proximal limb can be comfortably brought out to skin level, and the distal limb anastomosed directly to the renal pelvis (Fig. 2.2a). A variant is to make the stomal limb antiperistaltic by bringing out the distal ureter as the stoma and anastomosing the proximal ureter to it end-to-side (Fig. 2.2b). This

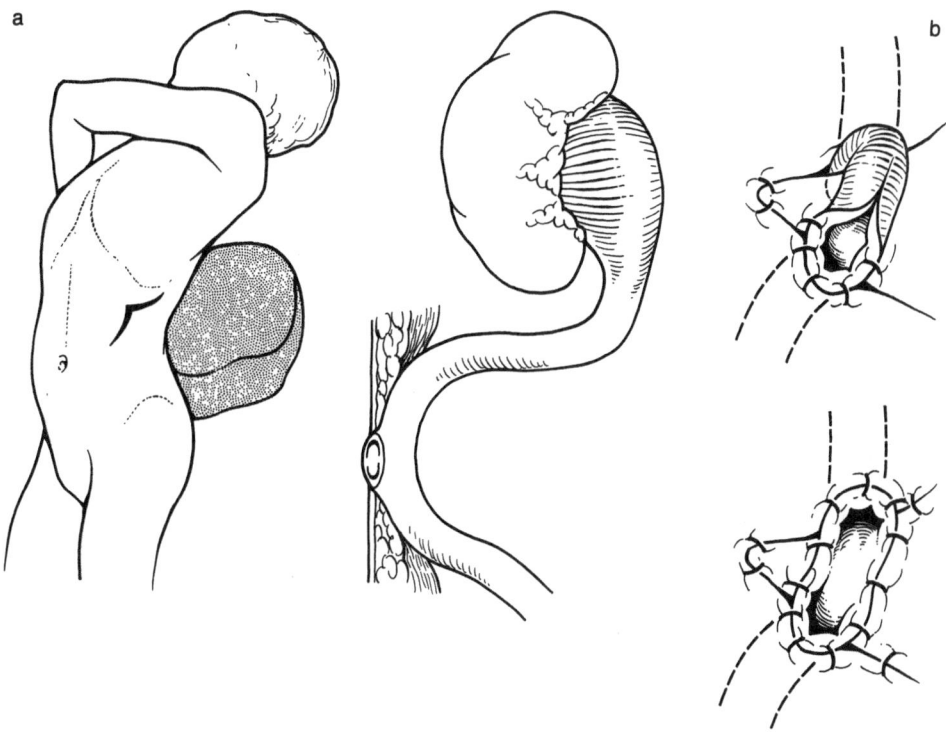

Fig.2.1. Loop ureterostomy. **a** Positioning and skin incision for high left loop ureterostomy. **b** Formation of the stoma.

alternative has been successfully employed in a small series of cases, both as a primary method of drainage and as part of a staged closure of loop ureterostomies (A. E. MacKinnon personal communication 1981). In the ring procedure the ureters at the base of the loop are anastomosed side-to-side with a stoma of some 1.5–2 cm diameter (Fig. 2.2c). If there is any element of pelvi-ureteric obstruction the distal limb can be anastomosed directly to the renal pelvis. The apex of the loop is brought out and opened in the usual way.

End Ureterostomy

The type chosen depends not only on whether the diversion is intended to be temporary or permanent, but also on the degree of dilatation of the two ureters. If both ureters are considerably dilated, it is preferable to bring both out at a single site rather than to have two widely separated stomas. A vogue existed for siting these double-barrelled stomas below the umbilicus in the midline; experience of a number of cases has convinced the author that this site is inherently unsatisfactory and if at all possible a conventional lateralised stoma is to be preferred, with the more dilated ureter brought across the midline (Fig. 2.3a) (Eckstein and Kapila 1970; Sweitzer and Kelalis 1978). In patients with unilateral disease, where total diversion is considered advisable, the affected ureter is brought out ipsilaterally to form the

a

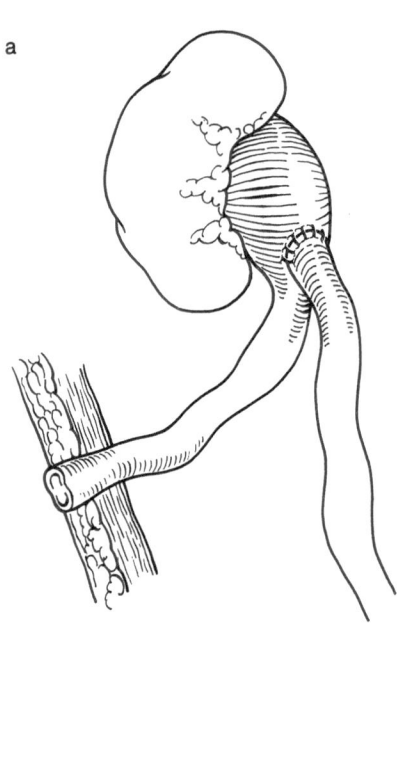

c

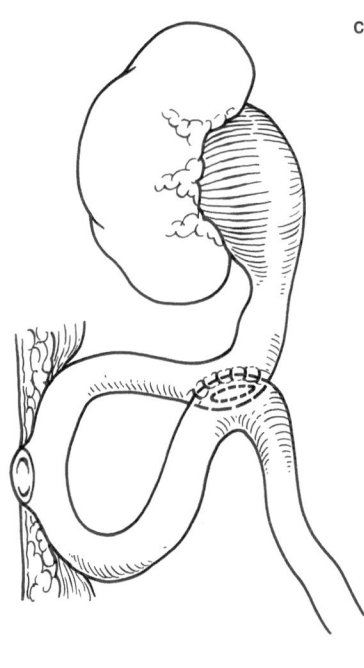

b

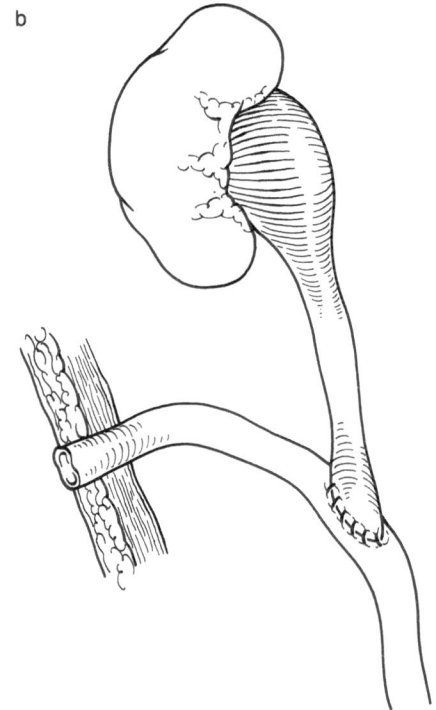

Fig.2.2. a Sober ureterostomy.
b 'Reversed' Sober ureterostomy. **c** Ring ureterostomy.

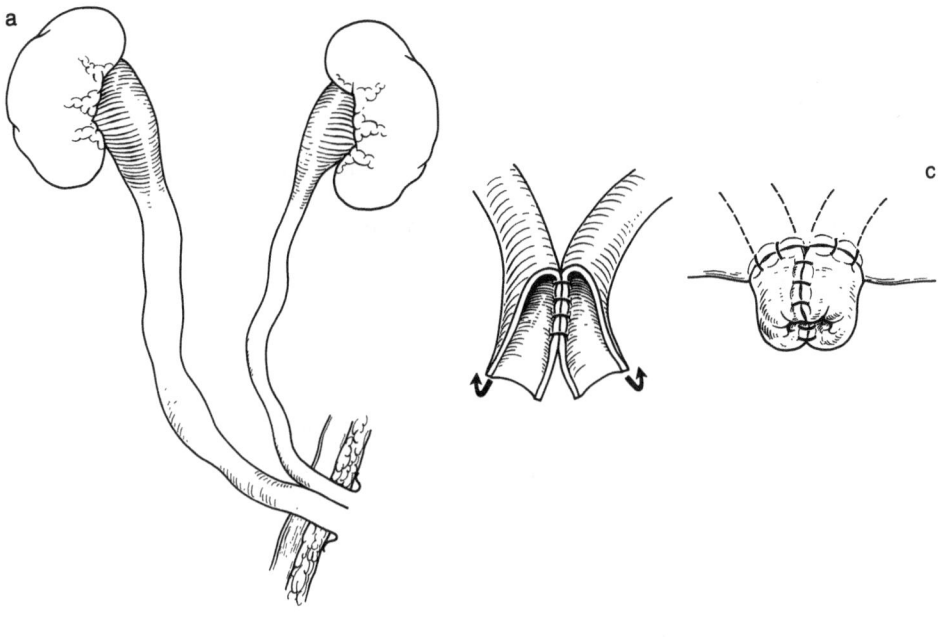

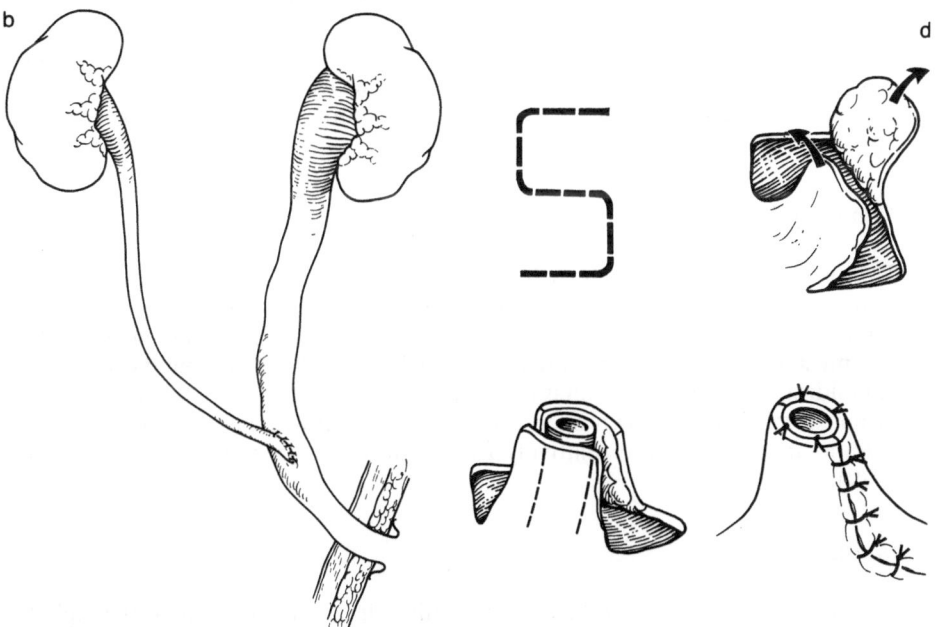

Fig. 2.3. End-ureterostomy. **a** Double-barrelled. The more dilated ureter is brought across the midline. **b** Transureteroureterostomy when one ureter is of normal calibre. The dilated ureter brought out ipsilaterally to form the stoma. **c** Method for forming a single conjoined stoma for double-barrelled ureterostomy. **d** Use of double skin flaps for surrounding a terminal ureterostomy when the ureter cannot be everted.

stoma and the opposite ureter is crossed over to it as a transureteroureterostomy (Fig. 2.3b).

If both ureters are being diverted, a transperitoneal approach is preferable to attempting an entirely extraperitoneal procedure; fears that this may result in adhesion intestinal obstruction have not materialised in our hands. The ureters are divided close to the bladder and mobilised proximally just enough to bring them in a smooth curve, extraperitoneally, to the chosen destination. For a transuretero-ureterostomy, the smaller ureter is spatulated for some 2 cm before being anastomosed end-to-side to the opposite ureter. The anastomosis should be drained extraperitoneally.

The stoma is usually formed by everting the ureter to give a 1–2 cm nipple. For a double-barrelled ureterostomy, the two ureters may be incised along their medial borders, joined together, and everted as a single stoma (Fig. 2.3c). To avoid stenosis at skin level, single (Fig. 2.3d) or double (q.v.) skin flaps can be incorporated in the stoma. When the ureter is too short or too narrow to be safely everted it may be surrounded by skin flaps.

Intestinal Conduits

Stoma Site

Special care is required in patients with congenital lesions of the cord in whom there is an actual or potential spinal deformity (Chap. 5). Otherwise in children, no special problems should be encountered in siting the stoma, provided that the usual precautions are taken to ensure that this is in an area which is flat or convex, standing and sitting, and that the appliance will not impinge on a bony prominence or operation scar. If a stomatherapist is available, which should certainly be the case in an institution performing any number of diversions, advice should be sought both pre- and post-operatively (Chap. 5).

Choice of Conduit

This is governed largely by whether it is intended this should be refluxing or non-refluxing. Although anti-refluxing uretero-ileal anastomoses are described, using a ureteric nipple (Turner-Warwick and Ashken 1967; Douglas 1979) or a seromuscular gutter (Itatani and Sonoda 1978), these have not found widespread use in children in whom the colon is preferred if ureteric reflux is to be prevented. Fears of anastomotic breakdown need not be a deterrent to a large bowel conduit since colonic anastomoses are relatively free of problems in children (Rickwood et al. 1979).

Incision

A transverse incision is preferred since this is less likely to dehisce (Campbell and Swenson 1972) and is unlikely to compromise any future stoma site should the initial one prove unsatisfactory. The incision is made some 3 cm above the pubis and the upper flap dissected off the rectus sheath for 3–4 cm. The sheath is incised transversely at this higher level and, in thin patients, continuation as a Pfannenstiel incision gives adequate access. In plump patients transverse division of the recti is advisable. Transverse incisions give relatively poor access to the intestinal mesentery and none to the upper ureters. A vertical incision is required if it is anticipated that one of the less conventional conduits (jejunal, transverse or descending colon) or a high ureteric anastomosis might be needed.

Isolation of the Conduit

The length should be kept to the minimum required to reach from the posterior abdominal wall to the stoma site, with a spout not exceeding 2 cm. It is customary to allow a little extra length and trim distally at the end of the procedure. For this reason, and for the purposes of any later revision of the stoma, the feeding vessels should be based towards the proximal end of the conduit and, in children, these need comprise only a single major artery and vein. For a high anastomosis to the urinary tract a conduit of transverse colon can be isolated on the middle colic and descending colon on the descending branch of the left colic artery.

Restoration of Intestinal Continuity

A practice exists among paediatric surgeons to anastomose intestine with a single layer of interrupted inverting sutures, but except in babies, a conventional two-layer anastomosis is more expeditious and equally satisfactory. The appendix is removed as a routine prophylactic measure.

Refluxing Ureterointestinal Anastomoses

Any of the usual methods is equally applicable to small bowel and colonic conduits and no particular method appears to possess any inherent superiority in terms of leakage or stricture. The commonly employed end-to-side anastomosis makes for easy identification of the ureters if revision is needed, but has the disadvantage that any leak is intraperitoneal and liable to lead to serious consequences (Kafetsioulis and Swinney 1968). The author's preference is for the Wallace II technique (Wallace 1970) (Fig. 2.4) which provides a long uretero-intestinal stoma which can be entirely covered by posterior peritoneum and drained extraperitoneally; any leak has been without serious consequence and has healed spontaneously.

In patients with massive hydronephrosis or with ureters that are considered unusable by virtue of atony or peri-ureteric fibrosis, a transverse colonic (Johnston 1974) or a jejunal or descending colonic conduit may be anastomosed directly to the renal pelvis.

Anti-Refluxing Uretero-Colic Anastomoses

The submucosal tunnel technique (Leadbetter and Clarke 1954) is well known but the Mathisen (1953) bud, which is especially applicable when the length of ureter available is somewhat short, merits some description (Fig. 2.5). A full thickness flap of colon is fashioned some 2 cm in length and of a width just a little greater than the ureteric circumference. The apex of the flap is sutured circumferentially around the spatulated end of the ureter with four interrupted sutures; it is an advantage to hold one of these as a stay until construction of the bud is complete. The remainder of the flap is sutured longitudinally around the distal ureter, the completed bud inverted

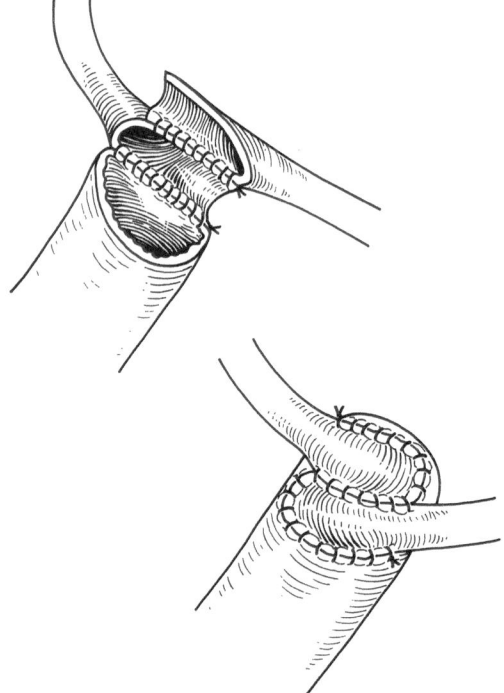

Fig.2.4. Wallace II uretero-ileal anastomosis.

into the lumen of the conduit and the colon closed over it in two layers. Absorbable sutures are used throughout. (There is much to be said for avoiding use of non-absorbable sutures anywhere in a conduit — stone formation is common enough after these procedures without further adding to the risk).

Whichever method is used, if the ureter is grossly dilated it will require trimming in its terminal 5 cm or so if reflux is to be prevented (Althausen et al. 1978). This is achieved by the Hendren (1972) technique (Fig. 2.6a–c). It is vital that the ureteric blood supply is carefully preserved; only the lateral portion of the ureter is excised sufficient to allow light closure over a 12 or 14F catheter. Watertight closure is obtained in two layers (inner, all ureteric layers, outer, peri-ureteric adventitial tissue) with continuous fine chromic catgut sutures.

Extra versus Trans-Peritoneal Conduits

The case for the former has been argued by Stevens and Eckstein (1977) who state the postoperative course is smoother and long-term complications less frequent. The case for the transperitoneal conduit is that (a) it is easier to perform; (b) problems with the vascular pedicle are less common (Stevens and Eckstein 1977); (c) postoperative intestinal obstruction is usually due to adhesions rather than internal hernia and the extraperitoneal conduit offers no advantage in this respect; (d) other studies have not demonstrated long term advantages for the extraperitoneal conduit (Cook et al. 1968; Pekarovič et al. 1968); and (e) any form of revisionary surgery is easier with a transperitoneal conduit.

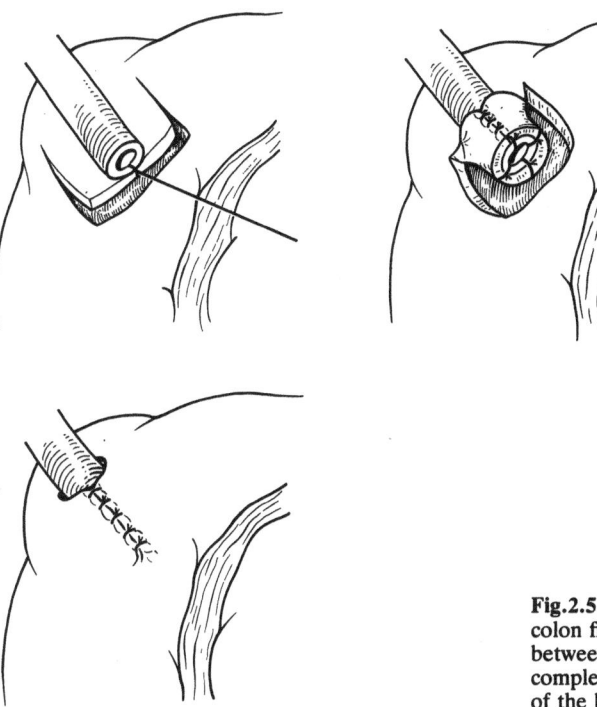

Fig.2.5. The Mathisen bud. *Top left*, the colon flap and placement of the first suture between ureter and flap. *Top right*, completion of the bud. *Bottom*, inversion of the bud and closure of the colon over it.

Formation of the Stoma

A spout of 2 cm is quite sufficient. McEwan and Clark (1973) suggest that function of the conduit and stoma is improved if the blood supply to its distal extremity is kept intact, rather than baring it of mesentery in its terminal 2–3 cm. Smith (1972) attempts to reduce the incidence of stomal stenosis by incorporating skin flaps (Fig. 2.7). It is unnecessary to excise triangular areas from the outer layer of the stoma to receive the flaps; after simple vertical incision of the outer layer, the edges part spontaneously at the base to provide the required shape.

Postoperative Drainage

It is advisable to perform ureteroileal anastomoses over splints — 6F or 8F infant feeding tubes or umbilical catheters serve very well — but the author has found no advantage in leaving these in situ postoperatively. On the other hand, external drainage of the anastomosis is always advisable.

Ureterosigmoidostomy in Continuity

(See Chap. 3)

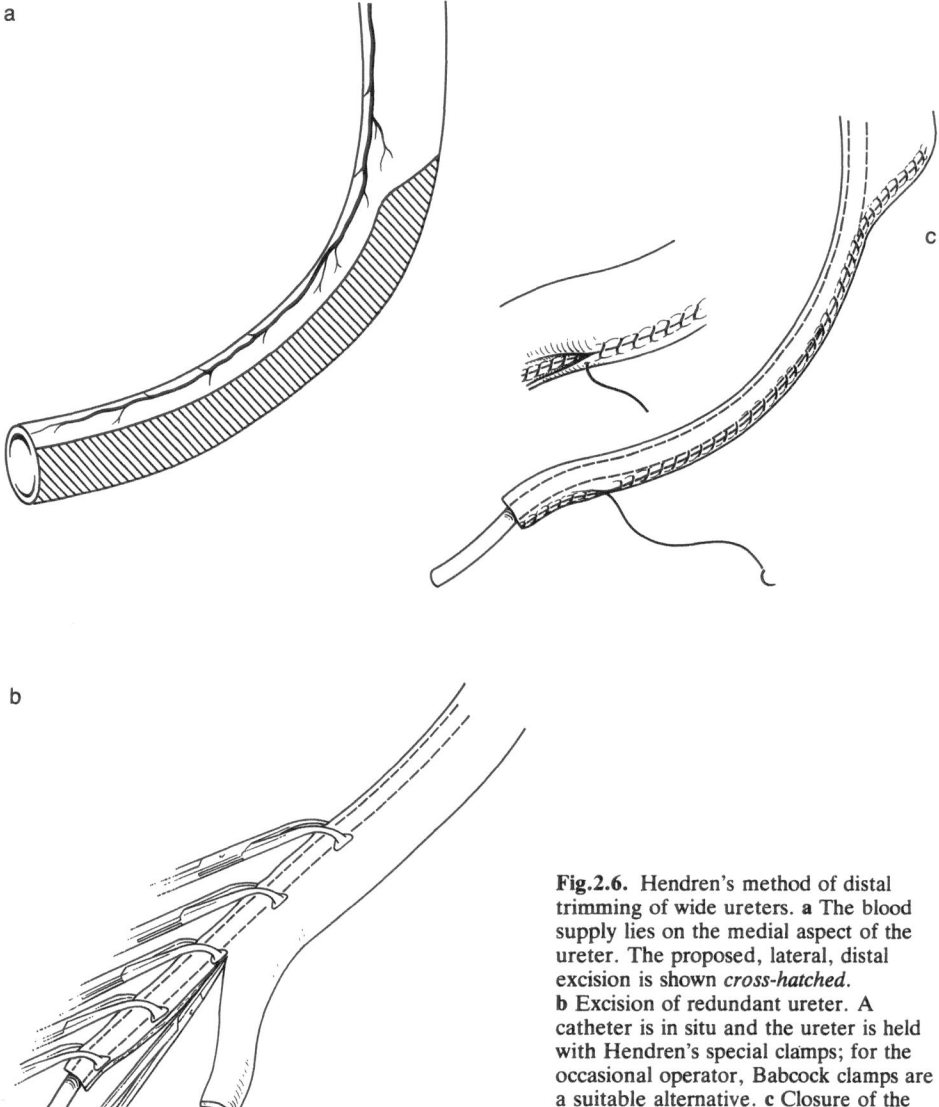

Fig.2.6. Hendren's method of distal trimming of wide ureters. **a** The blood supply lies on the medial aspect of the ureter. The proposed, lateral, distal excision is shown *cross-hatched*.
b Excision of redundant ureter. A catheter is in situ and the ureter is held with Hendren's special clamps; for the occasional operator, Babcock clamps are a suitable alternative. **c** Closure of the ureteric defect in two layers of running fine chromic catgut sutures.

Staged Ureterosigmoidostomy in Continuity (Hendren 1976)

The disadvantages of the one-stage procedure are that it must be delayed until the patient has good rectal control and that revision of the uretero-sigmoid anastomosis is not without hazard. An alternative is to construct a non-refluxing colonic conduit at about the age of 2 years. Any obstruction or reflux at the ureterosigmoid anastomosis (Hendren considers reflux occurring at a pressure of 35 cm of water or more can be ignored) is corrected prior to the second stage when the child has achieved good rectal control. The stoma is taken down and the distal end of the conduit anastomosed end-to-end to the sigmoid colon (Fig. 2.8a,b).

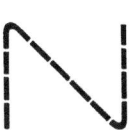
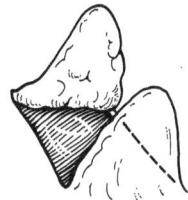

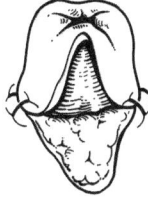
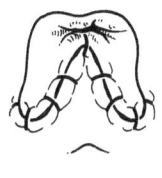

Fig. 2.7. Use of skin flaps to avoid stomal stenosis. *Top left*, skin incision. *Top right*, skin flaps raised. *Bottom left*, incision of the outer layer of the stoma prior to receiving the skin flap. *Bottom right*, skin flap sutured in position.

Vesical Diversions

Procedures

a) Suprapubic cystotomy

This calls for no special description whether it is performed as a procedure in its own right or as part of some other procedure. It is customary to use a latex Malecot catheter, 14F for babies and up to 18F for older children.

b) Tubeless vesicostomy (Blocksum 1957)

The bladder is approached through a midline lower abdominal incision and opened anteriorly by a stab incision. It is then mobilised sufficiently to enable the wall to be sutured to the rectus sheath, and the aperture to be marsupialised to the surrounding skin. The stoma should admit an index finger.

c) Tube vesicostomy (Lapides et al. 1960)

The bladder is first filled with saline. For adults each side of the bladder and skin flaps measures 4 and 2.5 cm respectively, and these dimensions need to be scaled down appropriately for children (Fig. 2.9a). The four corners of the bladder flap should be marked with stay sutures before the flap is cut. The skin flap incorporates the full thickness of subcutaneous fat. When cutting the aperture in the anterior rectus sheath, the sheath should be drawn down to its original level in the lower incision in order to avoid kinking in the channel between bladder and skin. The two flaps are sutured together to form a tube with a single layer of 2–O or 3–O absorbable sutures, while any distal defect in the bladder is closed in two layers (Fig. 2.9b). It is recommended that the bladder should be drained by a transurethral or suprapubic catheter for two weeks postoperatively.

If tubeless vesicostomy is intended as a permanent diversion, it will be necessary to obliterate the bladder outlet if there is an appreciable degree of detrusor instability or sphincter weakness incontinence (Chap. 1).

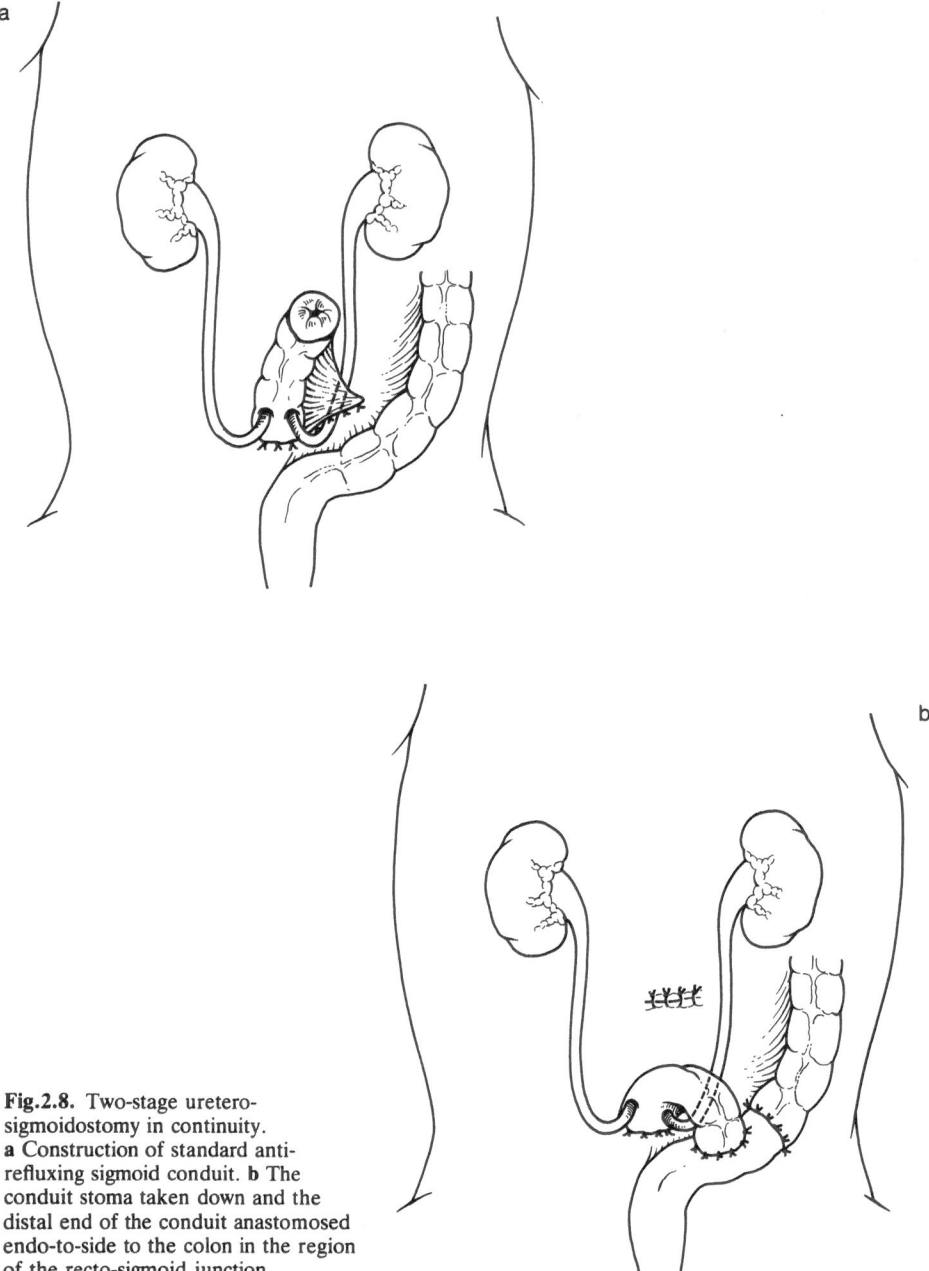

Fig.2.8. Two-stage ureterosigmoidostomy in continuity.
a Construction of standard anti-
refluxing sigmoid conduit. **b** The
conduit stoma taken down and the
distal end of the conduit anastomosed
endo-to-side to the colon in the region
of the recto-sigmoid junction.

Indications

a) Simple suprapubic cystotomy is widely used in children for short-term drainage
in any procedure where the bladder has been opened, and for this purpose proves
more reliable and less troublesome than a urethral catheter. The catheter can usually
be safely removed one week postoperatively.

a

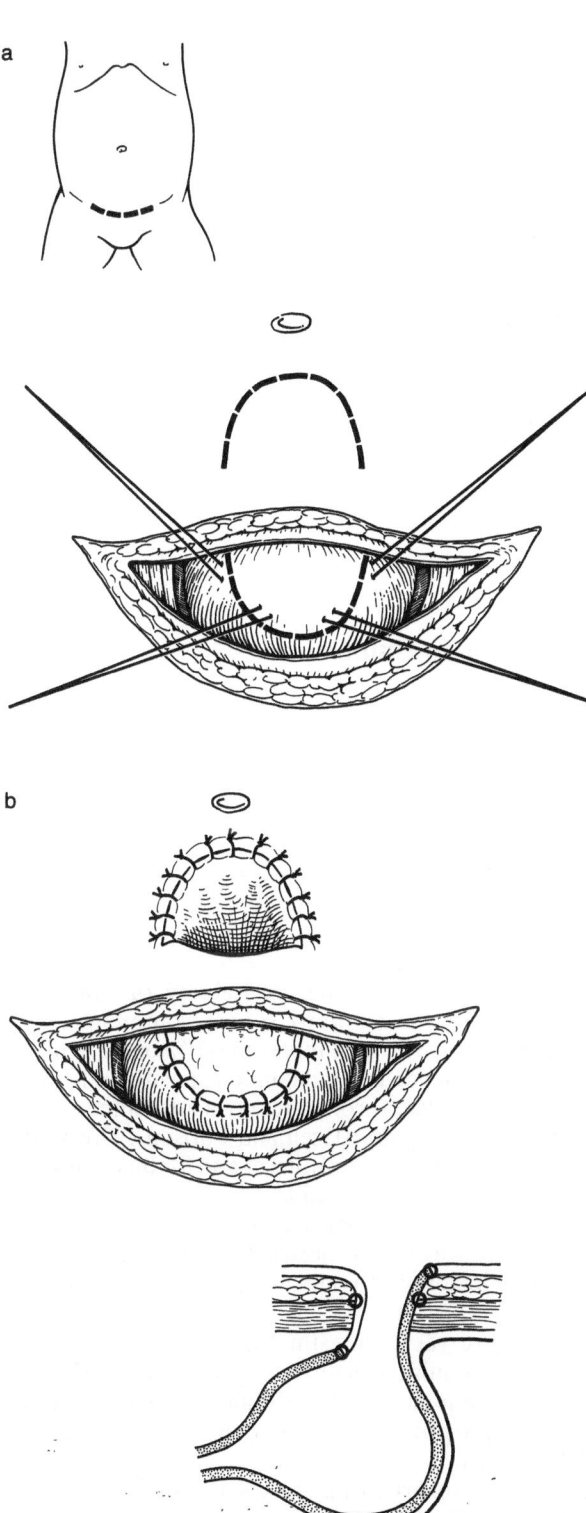

b

Fig.2.9. Lapides tubeless
vesicostomy. **a** Pfannenstiel incision
for exposure of the bladder. The
corners of the bladder flap are
marked by stay sutures. The
inverted 'U' skin flap is also shown.
b The skin and bladder flaps
transposed to form the vesico-
cutaneous conduit.

b) Tubeless vesicostomy continues to enjoy some popularity in the United States as a medium-term measure in infants and children with infra-vesical obstruction, especially those with neuro-vesical dysfunction (Allen 1980; Bruce and Gonzales 1980). The advantages lie in its being a relatively minor procedure and one which can be easily reversed. The disadvantages are several (Bell et al. 1968). The stoma site is not ideal and is positively unsatisfactory in the presence of lordosis. Stomal stenosis, symptomatic bacteriuria and calculus formation are not uncommon. Most importantly, the procedure may fail in its principal object of promoting good drainage of the bladder. For these reasons tubeless vesicostomy has seen little use in children in the United Kingdom; with neurovesical dysfunction alternative methods of promoting bladder emptying exist which are more effective and less prone to complication (Chap. 1).

As a permanent urinary diversion for children, vesicostomy would seem to have very little to recommend it.

Indications for Urinary Diversion in Children

Neuro-Vesical Dysfunction

(See Chap. 1).

Congenital Anomalies Associated with Urinary Incontinence

Bladder Extrophy and Variants

It is still possible to hold extreme views as to the desirability or otherwise of aggressive reconstructive surgery in an attempt to secure continence *per via naturalis*, but a middle of the road approach accepts that some 40% of these bladders are so small that reconstruction could never give adequate capacity and for these diversion is unavoidable. For the remainder, reconstruction is attempted accepting that only around a third become adequately dry (Ezell and Carlson 1970; Williams 1972; Williams and Keeton 1973). For girls who are still wet and for boys who cannot be managed by a penile appliance, diversion is advisable.

Provided that rectal control is good and the upper renal tracts are normal (which is usually the case except in a few instances where obstruction or reflux supervenes after reconstruction), ureterosigmoidostomy as a one- or two-stage procedure is the diversion of choice.

In the much rarer and more severe vesico-intestinal fissure (cloacal extrophy) anomaly, surviving patients usually require faecal (ileostomy) and urinary (ileal conduit) diversion. If the colon is of adequate length and diameter, it may be isolated as a mucous fistula at the initial neonatal procedure and later used for a non-refluxing conduit (Sukarochana and Sicker 1978).

Urinary diversion is held as a last resort in patients with epispadias who are incontinent since the results of reconstructive procedures on the bladder neck are much more encouraging in this group (Leadbetter 1964).

Ectopic Ureters

Diversion need normally be considered only for the unusual condition of bilateral single ectopic ureters (Mogg 1974), in which the bladder neck is always incompetent. If one or both upper tracts are reasonably normal, ureteric reimplantation and bladder outlet reconstruction may be attempted (Williams and Lightwood 1972; Williams and Snyder 1976). However an ectopic ureter is usually characterised by a degree of congenital dysplasia affecting also the kidney which it drains and for a proportion of patients with bilateral single ectopic ureters, permanent abdominal wall diversion is the safer means of securing dryness.

Urogenital Sinus and Cloaca

In the more severe forms there is high confluence between urethra and vagina, a short or absent urethra and an incompetent or absent bladder neck, leading to either stress or total urinary incontinence (Williams and Bloomberg 1976). In cloaca there is an anorectal anomaly, in the form of a recto-vaginal fistula, in addition to the urogenital sinus anomaly. The situation is further complicated by an appreciable incidence of congenital upper tract anomalies, including bilateral single ectopic ureters, and in cloaca there may also be a sacral deficiency with a corresponding neurological deficit. Finally there is not infrequently an element of stenosis of the single perineal opening with pooling of urine in the vagina causing an obstructive uropathy (Hendren 1980).

At one time it was considered that the more severely affected patients would be irretrievably incontinent and permanent urinary diversion unavoidable. Reconstructive procedures now exist (Williams and Snyder 1976; Hendren 1980) which offer a reasonable prospect of achieving urinary control and which take precedence over permanent urinary diversion in patients whose upper tracts are in reasonably good shape.

Pelvic Malignant Disease

For practical purposes this means rhabdomyosarcoma, prostate in boys, vagina and uterus in girls and bladder in either sex. Until recently treatment comprised radiotherapy plus anterior exenteration with permanent urinary diversion. The results were wretched. The advent of aggressive chemotherapy has greatly improved the outlook for this disease (Malpas et al. 1976) and patients have been successfully treated without recourse to radical surgery. The role of surgery is currently in some doubt (Gornall et al. 1979; Neifield et al. 1979) and patients with this tumour are always best referred to centres specialising in paediatric oncology.

Megaureters

To the surgeon with only occasional contact with paediatric urological problems, the dramatic radiological appearance of the megaureter would seem to cry out for a diversionary procedure. This would be a grave mistake. Not only are better alternatives usually available but diversion may fail to effect any improvement. Full discussion of this large and still controversial topic is beyond the scope of this chapter, but consideration of some basic principles may help to put the role of diversion in perspective (Table 2.1).

Table 2.1. Classification of megaureter

Obstructed megaureter	*Primary*—Primary obstructed megaureter —Ureterocele —Iatrogenic (post-reimplantation)
	Secondary—Posterior urethral valves (infra-vesical—Neuro-vesical dysfunction obstruction)
Refluxing megaureter	*Primary*—Primary refluxing megaureter (megaureter/megacystis syndrome
	Secondary—Posterior urethral valves (infra-vesical—Neuro-vesical dysfunction obstruction)
Non-obstructed/ non-refluxing megaureter	*Primary*—Congenital dysplasia (prune belly syndrome, ectopic ureters)
	Secondary—Polyuric states —Iatrogenic (following reconstructive surgery)

Histological Studies

Emery and Gill (1974) identified two types of megaureter, one with an appreciable increase in the muscle bulk (hyperplasia, hypertrophy or both) along with an increased connective tissue content, the other without any such increase. It was suggested that the first is a partially compensated ureter in which recovery of useful peristaltic function is possible, the second a decompensated ureter incapable of recovery of function.

In a combined light and electron microscopic study (Hanna et al. 1977a), three appearances were described, corresponding clinically with the obstructed, the refluxing and the dysplastic megaureter, and a small series (Hanna et al. 1977b) suggested that consideration of both the morphology and ultrastructure of the ureteric smooth muscle cells provided a guide to the likely response to surgery.

Investigations

Ordinary radiological studies have proved unreliable in distinguishing the obstructed from the unobstructed megaureter and can now be supplemented by pressure/ perfusion studies (Whitaker 1973, 1979) diuresis renography (O'Reilly et al. 1978), and radioactive isotope transit times (Whitfield et al. 1978). In some cases uretero-vesical obstruction is only evident with a full bladder (Whitfield et al. 1976). Although these techniques hold promise it is perhaps too early to judge how far they will improve the quality of treatment.

Treatment

The distinction between the various types of function in megaureters is of great importance in treatment. In general terms the obstructed megaureter responds well to surgery, including diversion, whilst the non-obstructed, and especially the dysplastic ureter responds poorly. The obstructed megaureter is, however, usually best managed by removal of the cause of the obstruction, with diversion reserved for a minority of cases which fall into two general categories.

1) Infants with severe bilateral disease, presenting with uraemia, severe electrolyte imbalance and often urinary infection with septicaemia. This is most commonly seen in posterior urethral valves, but may occur with any form of obstructive megaureter. Immediate management consists in correction of electrolyte imbalance (and even peritoneal dialysis) and antibiotic therapy for infection (Johnston and Kulatilake 1972). Many patients improve sufficiently on this regime to allow early correction of the obstruction. Improved medical management of the uraemic, septicaemic infant would seem to have materially reduced the need for diversion (Williams et al. 1973), which is now reserved for cases where sastisfactory improvement has not occurred after 24–48 hours' treatment (Rabinowitz et al. 1977) and is more often needed in the presence of infection. The choice lies between nephrostomy or high ureterostomy (loop, Sober or ring) and calls for fine judgement. The former is best avoided if it is thought that diversion will be required for more than a few weeks.

2) Where upper tract dilatation does not improve, or even deteriorates, after the cause of the obstruction has been removed (Johnston and Kulatilake 1971; Williams et al. 1973; Rabinowitz et al. 1979a). It is in these cases that the antegrade pressure/perfusion test is of especial value in detecting residual uretero-vesical obstruction (Whitaker 1973, 1979; Whitfield et al. 1976), which, if present, may respond to ureteric reimplantation with or without a covering high ureterostomy or nephrostomy depending on the quality of renal function. There remains a small residuum of patients with bilateral obstructive megaureters who fail to respond to adequate surgical treatment (Williams and Hulme Moir 1970; Johnston and Kulatilake 1971; Williams et al. 1973; Rabinowitz et al. 1979a,b) for whom permanent diversion, usually end ureterostomy, is unavoidable, and which may serve only to stabilise rather than improve renal function.

The place for diversion for the non-obstructed megaureter would seem even less. When secondary to bladder outlet obstruction severe examples are usually associated with poor and irrecoverable renal function; even high diversion in these circumstances is of little more than prognostic value. Less severe examples, whether secondary to urethral valves or neurogenic dysfunction, may be improved by diversion, but usually respond equally well, or better, if attention is directed solely to relieving outlet obstruction (Johnston and Kulatilake 1971; Philp and Rickwood 1981). A few neonates with prune belly syndrome present as an acute emergency and respond to a high temporary ureterostomy (Barnhouse 1972; Williams and Parker 1974). In most patients with this condition surgical interference with the upper renal tracts is best avoided (Woodhouse et al. 1979); if there is an element of bladder outlet obstruction (Snyder et al. 1976) ureteric dilatation often improves after internal urethrotomy. The primary refluxing megaureter has generally proved a particularly poor candidate for surgery. Good results reported from extensive ureteric tailoring and reimplantation (Hendren 1972) have not been repeated in other series

(Johnston and Farkas 1975), and in the author's experience no useful advantage is ever gained by any form of diversion.

Urinary Diversion and Renal Transplantation

Despite every endeavour, a few children with obstructive or reflux uropathy will inevitably progress to renal failure and then the question of transplantation will arise. There is a natural reluctance to transplant into a bladder of unknown or dubious function and this aspect should not be forgotten in children who have undergone total diversion.

It is possible to transplant into intestinal conduits, but the number performed has been small and the results not especially encouraging (Castro et al. 1975; Firlit and Merkel 1977).

Complications and Results of Diversion in Children

Short-Term

Nephrostomy and loop ureterostomy are largely free of early complication except in the event of technical failure. Ureterostomies in which the ureter has been divided are prone to distal ischaemic necrosis which may necessitate semi-emergency conversion to a conduit diversion. The early complications of conduit diversions in children do not differ from those in adults but are less prevalent. All reports agree that the early post-operative mortality is low. At the Sheffield Children's Hospital there have been no such deaths for 15 years during which period 186 conduits have been performed.

Long-Term Surveillance after Diversion

As will be seen, no child who has undergone urinary diversion is ever free of risk of developing serious complications. Since these are usually asymptomatic in their retrievable stages, continuous and proper urological surveillance is essential and it is equally important that this is continued when the patient is passed on to an adult unit. A suggested scheme follows.

1) *Intravenous Pyelography*

The prime concern is always for the state of the upper renal tracts and the intravenous urogram remains the principal investigation in this respect. It is performed at 3 months after diversion (or any revisionary procedure) and, if all is well, again at 18 months and then at 2–5 year intervals depending on what is known of the state of the upper tracts and the function of the conduit. Such a scheme, designed to minimise exposure to radiation, is somewhat arbitrary, and bound on occasion to miss significant upper tract deterioration for some period of time. It is probable that use of ultrasound and isotope examinations will prove an invaluable means of keeping a closer watch on the condition of the upper tracts.

2) *Collection of Urine Specimens*

Faecal organisms abound on the stoma and in the terminal reaches of a conduit. They are far less prevalent in the depths of a conduit, the only site where their presence is significant. It is essential that specimens for bacteriological examination are collected from this and no other site (Bishop et al. 1971). The double lumen catheter is ideal, but for routine use, a single catheter technique is simpler and provides comparable results. After cleaning the stoma with saline, an 8FG to 10FG infant feeding tube is passed into the depths of the conduit. The first few drops of urine obtained are discarded and the remainder collected for bacteriological study. Only pure growths of an organism with a colony count of 10^5 organisms per ml or more are regarded as significant. How often this examination is required depends on the patient's 'form', but should not exceed 6-monthly intervals. Similar techniques and considerations apply to ureterostomies.

As important as bacteriological study is measurement of conduit residual urine on each occasion a specimen is taken. A sudden increase in residual may prompt investigation of the upper tracts (Fig. 2.10a,b).

3) *Loopograms*

The principle of this examination is simple but the interpretation sometimes less so; the surgeon will often gain useful extra information by being present at the study. A normal examination shows a short undilated conduit with active propulsive peristalsis, and free ureteric reflux (in refluxing conduits). A delayed film at 30 min should show complete clearance of contrast from the system. Two errors of interpretation are common. One is the assumption that poor drainage of the conduit is always due to stomal stenosis, but it may also be due to conduit malfunction (q.v.). The other is the belief that reflux excludes uretero-conduit obstruction; an example of this fallacy is shown in Fig. 2.11a,b.

Loopography is indicated

a) To determine the cause of any upper tract deterioration found on intravenous urogram.

b) To determine conduit function when significant residual urine is detected.

c) To confirm the effectiveness of anti-refluxing anastomoses; in such examinations the pressure at which any reflux is induced should be recorded (Hendren 1976).

d) To determine the length of conduit available if lengthening or resiting the stoma is contemplated.

4) *Electrolyte Measurements*

These are of limited value. Electrolyte imbalance is exceptional in children following conduit procedures except where the conduit has been constructed far too long (Smith 1972) or the renal function is already severely compromised (Kafetsioulis and Swinney 1968; Castro and Ram 1970). A rise in blood urea or creatinine should seldom be the first sign of upper tract problems; in children these values lie well within the normal range until there is gross upper tract dilatation, an event which should have been detected long before under the scheme outlined.

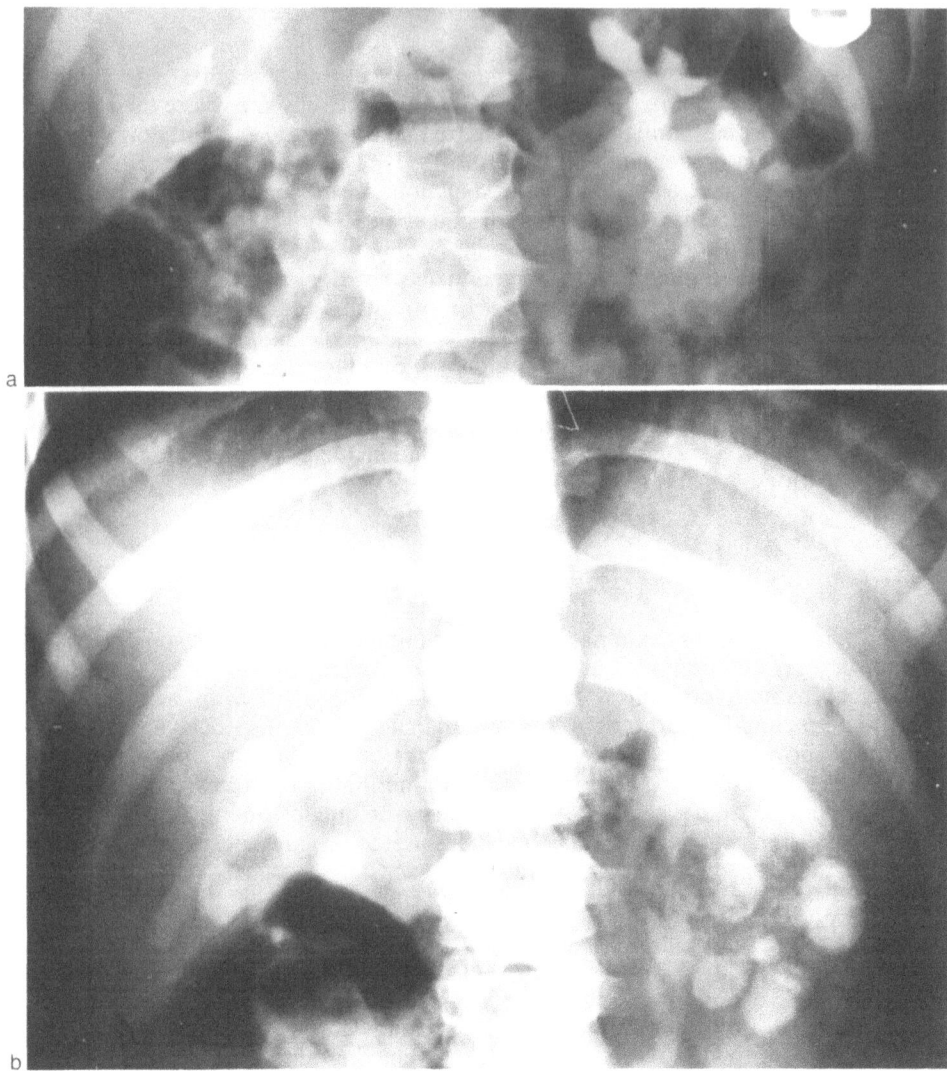

Fig.2.10. a I.V.P. 6 years following ileal conduit, showing mild upper tract dilatation. The conduit residual urine at this time was 25 ml. **b** I.V.P. 1 year later showing severe upper tract dilatation. The patient was asymptomatic but a conduit residual of 150 ml was considered sufficient reason for repeating the I.V.P.

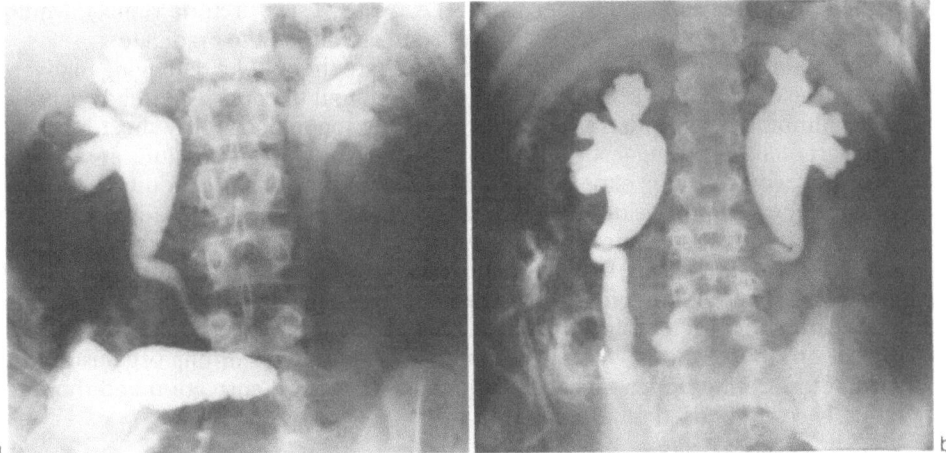

Fig.2.11. a Loopogram during filling showing ureteric reflux, and a dilated conduit with apparent outlet stenosis. The appearances of the conduit are in fact due to the radiologist having to inject contrast under pressure to demonstrate reflux. **b** 5-min drainage film showing complete clearance of contrast from the conduit but retention of contrast in the upper tracts. At operation tight bilateral uretero-ileal strictures were found.

Long-Term Complications and Management

Pyocystis

This irritating problem is largely confined to females of whom rather more than half suffer in some degree after diversion. It has a natural tendency to regress and is rarely a problem in teenagers and adults. Most cases respond to simple conservative measures. Systemic antibiotics as treatment or prophylaxis are of no value. Effective treatment consists of saline bladder lavage usually given daily for 5 days and weekly for a month. It is customary, but probably unnecessary, to add an antibiotic or an antiseptic (Noxytiolin, Hibitane) to the lavage. Surgery need only be considered for the few patients who do not respond or develop multiple recurrences and consists either of cystectomy or the lesser procedure of vaginal vesicostomy (Stevens and Eckstein 1975). It is worth bearing in mind that the former renders undiversion an impossible, and the latter a difficult, proposition.

Urinary Infection

It is common experience that even with adequate sampling techniques, an appreciable number of children have episodes of bacteriuria after diversion and their number may perhaps be increased by reflux of organisms from collecting bag to conduit (Bergman et al. 1977). Only a few episodes are symptomatic and need treatment on that account. In general terms, two patterns of infection are seen after diversion. The first is in patients with normal upper tracts and no evidence of supravesical infection preoperatively. Provided the system continues to function well, urinary infections are exceptional and an episode is often an early warning sign of deterioration of upper tracts or conduit function. The second follows diversion of dilated and often infected upper tracts (i.e., with vesico-ureteric reflux). Multiple urinary infections continue after diversion and are difficult to eradicate.

The main question, whether these infections are themselves damaging to diverted upper tracts, or merely serve, at worst, to compound the damage already caused by bad 'plumbing', has eluded a definitive answer, although one fairly short-term study (Stewart et al. 1979) suggests that most infections in refluxing conduits are harmless. The same would also be expected of satisfactory anti-refluxing conduits. In any large practice there are considerable logistic problems involved in maintaining sterile urines by frequent specimens and repeated courses of antibiotics, while attempts to achieve the same result by continuous chemoprophylaxis are not conspicuously successful. There is something to be said for concentrating attention on patients in whom infections are considered to be a hazard, namely those with a history of stone formation, those who have repeated infections with urea-splitting organisms, those with deteriorating upper tracts not amenable to surgical correction and those with severely compromised renal function.

Stomal Problems

Problems with appliance fitting (Chap. 5) cannot be divorced from problems with the stoma itself. The finding on a domiciliary study of spina bifida patients (Woodburn 1973) that only 10% were free of stomal or appliance problems indicates that these are much commoner than the medical literature suggests. The statement that 'a healthy looking stoma which shows active peristalsis is a reliable sign of a healthy and active conduit' (McEwan and Clark 1973) may possess some general validity, but with children is too riddled with exceptions to be a useful guide.

a) Stomal retraction
A flat stoma may occur spontaneously or more commonly after an inadequate revision. Provided the site is satisfactory, appliance fitting is usually no problem, but the phenomenon may convert an indifferent site into one which is quite unsatisfactory. A flat stoma is not necessarily associated with stenosis or conduit malfunction.

b) Encrustation
Although undoubtedly much less common with modern appliances, this problem still occurs and is by no means always due to bad management. For reasons unknown it frequently responds dramatically to Penicillin-V in low dosage, 125 mg/day.

c) Stomal stenosis
Loop ureterostomies are almost free of this complication. Stenosis in end-ureterostomies is often described as affecting only the stoma, but not infrequently involves the entire distal ureter as it passes through the abdominal wall. It is to be admitted that attempts to retrieve this situation by excising the stenotic length and reforming the stoma or converting to a conduit, have met with little success. Unlike conduits, ureterostomy stenosis may respond to dilatation.

With the exception of Smith (1972), who incorporates skin flaps in the stoma, stenosis is reported as a common complication after conduit diversion in childhood (Ray and de Dominico 1972; Scott 1973; Middleton and Hendren 1976; Stevens and Eckstein 1977; Dunn et al. 1979; Elder et al. 1979; Pitts and Muecke 1979). Unfortunately there is no precise definition of the term, and it is often mistakenly assumed that stomal stenosis and an increased residual urine go hand in hand, but it is not hard to find stomas scarcely accepting an 8FG catheter, but with low conduit residual and satisfactory upper tracts, and this situation may persist for years if not indefinitely. Conversely there exist stomas readily accepting an index finger, but with large conduit residuals and upper tracts suffering correspondingly. Management of stomal stenosis must be considered in the context of conduit function as a whole and is dealt with under that heading.

It remains to be stated that the stenosis almost always lies at skin level, and although the problem may be more prevalent in the earlier years after diversion (Stevens and Eckstein 1977), fresh examples continue to present at our unit many years postoperatively.

In a recent very comprehensive review of the technical aspects of urological stomas, Bloom et al. (1981) favour a variation of Turnbull's loop or knuckle stoma in ileal conduits, particularly in obese patients. They report fewer post-operative complications with loop compared with bud or end stomas and in particular have not had any stomal stenosis.

Conduit Malfunction

A satisfactory conduit expeditiously expels its contents by active, propulsive peristalsis. Even in the absence of organic stomal stenosis, with the passage of time an increasing number of conduits fail to empty effectively. Three types of activity in conduits have been described: active propulsive peristalsis, churning non-propulsive peristalsis, and complete atony (Kafetsioulis and Swinney 1970). The churning type was sometimes, and the atonic type always, associated with delayed emptying of the conduit. Increased residual urine may therefore be due to outlet obstruction or malfunction of the conduit or both. Attempts to differentiate these factors by conduit pressure studies (Pekarovič et al. 1968; Mogg and Syme 1969; Magnus 1977) have not found a place in routine practice, where a combination of measurement of residual urine and floroscopy of the conduit usually provides sufficient information on which to base treatment.

It is, of course, primarily when there is reflux, that conduit stasis is liable to lead to upper tract deterioration, although severe degrees may lead to problems even when reflux has been prevented.

A conduit residual of less than 5 ml is ideal, and 5–25 ml acceptable provided the upper tracts are stable. A value over 25 ml is usually an indication for further study; if there is active peristalsis in the conduit a good response can be anticipated from revision of the stoma even if it does not appear to be particularly narrowed (Fig. 2.12a–c). A conduit showing poor or absent peristalsis does not usually recover useful function no matter how wide the stoma can be made nor however much it is shortened. Such conduits may also be associated with atonic ureters (Fig. 2.13), but if ureteric peristalsis remains active, substitution of a new conduit may improve the condition of the upper tracts (Fig. 2.14a,b).

Because stoma revision is such a common procedure a few technical details are given. Laparotomy is only needed when extensive mobilisation of the conduit is required to gain sufficient length to form a new stoma. Ordinarily the stoma is circumcised some 2 mm from the mucocutaneous junction and the incision deepened around the conduit into the peritoneal cavity, where by division of adhesions surrounding the conduit and its mesentery, sufficient length can be obtained to reform the stoma. The conduit and mesentery are divided just proximal to the stenosis (or more proximally if the conduit is especially redundant). The deep layers are closed around the conduit which is everted to form the new stoma. The

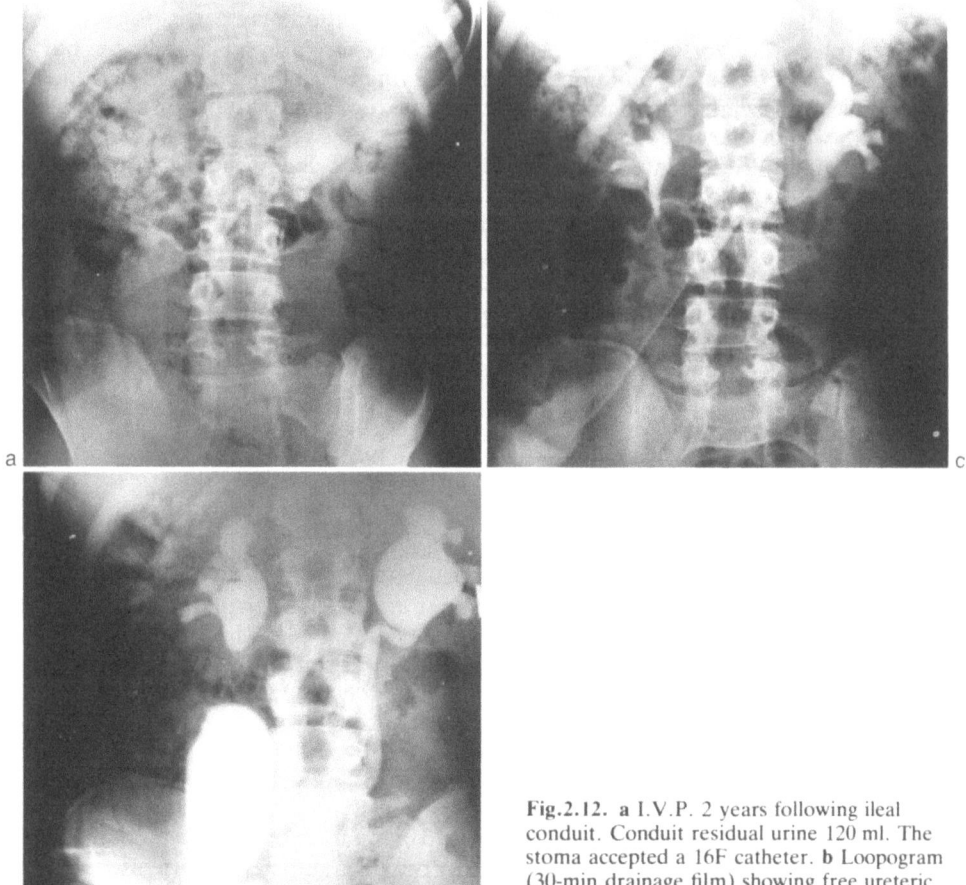

Fig.2.12. **a** I.V.P. 2 years following ileal conduit. Conduit residual urine 120 ml. The stoma accepted a 16F catheter. **b** Loopogram (30-min drainage film) showing free ureteric reflux and poor drainage from a conduit which is dilated and redundant but showing good peristalsis. **c** I.V.P. 4 months after stoma revision, showing marked upper renal tracts. The conduit residual was 15 ml.

surrounding skin is usually scarred and simple resuture to the stoma invites further stenosis, a possibility which can be lessened either by excising the scar tissue and closing the resulting skin defect by a spiral advancement flap (David 1976), or by incorporating two or three 'Z' plastys around the mucocutaneous junction (Fig. 2.15).

On occasion sufficient conduit cannot be mobilised to form an everted stoma. A flat stoma is acceptable at a good site, but liable to lead to appliance problems at an indifferent site. In this circumstance it will be necessary either to 'add on' (Poor et al. 1975), or perhaps better, to construct a new conduit. In patients with a progressive spinal deformity, it is not uncommon to find the original stoma site becoming impossible to manage. If a suitable alternative exists it is usually possible to mobilise the conduit to this new site.

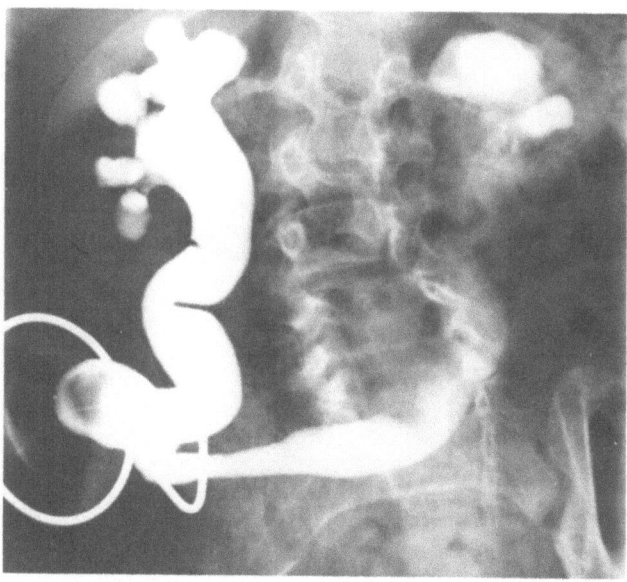

Fig.2.13. Loopogram (20-min drainage film) 11 years after construction of ileal conduit. The stoma had been revised and the conduit shortened on five previous occasions. The stoma accepts a 20F catheter, the conduit is short and there is free ureteric reflux. Despite this there is negligible drainage of contrast, with both ureters and conduit being completely aperistaltic.

Ileal Conduit Stenosis

This uncommon condition, of unknown aetiology, is characterised by chronic inflammation and fibrosis in the submucosal layer. It can occur many years after diversion (Mitchell et al. 1977) and may involve the whole (Fig. 2.16) or only part of the conduit. The stoma appears quite normal. Construction of a new conduit is usually required.

Ureteric Complications

a) Ureteroconduit stenosis
The reported incidence varies between 3% (Smith 1972) and 22% (Elder et al. 1979). It occurs both with refluxing and non-refluxing anastomoses (Althausen et al. 1978) and may be detected early, where the cause is likely to be technical failure, or late, where the cause is unknown. The author has encountered three late examples (5–14 years post diversion) in the last year. Provided ureteric peristalsis is satisfactory, response to surgical revision of the anastomosis is usually good.

b) Atonic ureters
Not all dilated ureters which follow diversion are obstructed. A proportion are observed at fluoroscopy to be quite atonic, and it is doubtful if anything can be done to retrieve this situation.

Urolithiasis

The reported incidence in long-term studies in children is 9% in ureterostomies (Rickwood 1978), 4% (Stevens and Eckstein 1977) to 12% (Dunn et al. 1979) in refluxing, and 4% (Althausen et al. 1978) to 16% (Elder et al. 1979) in anti-refluxing

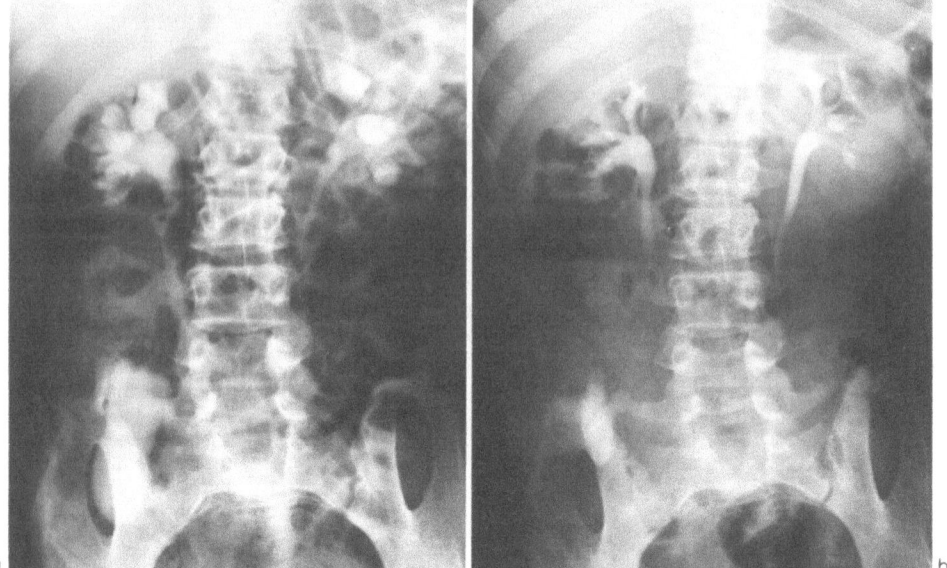

Fig.2.14. a I.V.P. 10 years following ileal conduit showing moderate upper tract dilatation. Three previous stoma revisions had failed to effect any improvement. Fluoroscopy showed the conduit to be aperistaltic but ureteric peristalsis was normal. **b** I.V.P. 6 months after construction of a new ileal conduit showing complete resolution of upper tract dilatation.

conduits. The stones are almost invariably of the mixed type associated with infection, and the two features common to almost all cases are dilated upper tracts and multiple infections with urea-splitting organisms. They are usually renal. Some remain small and solitary for years, but more often there is rapid progression to multiple and staghorn calculi.

It is difficult to give firm guidelines for management. Obstructive stones clearly require removal. Enthusiasm for intervention in other cases is tempered by the knowledge that the recurrence rate is high even after complete clearance and vigorous attempts to maintain sterile urine. On the other hand, renal function has been completely lost in the presence of multiple but seemingly non-obstructive calculi. One can only take shelter in the cliché that each case must be treated on its own merits.

The End Results of Diversion on the Upper Renal Tracts

Ureterostomies

Because of relatively small numbers, the variety of ureterostomies and the nature of the indications for which they are performed, it is difficult to comment in any detail on performance of this form of diversion. The general impression gained is that provided the ureter is capable of recovery of function, the medium and long-term results are neither better nor worse than those obtained with refluxing conduits (Lister et al. 1968; Sadlowski et al. 1978).

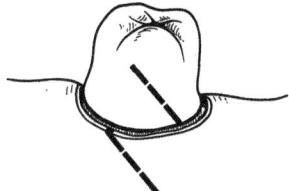

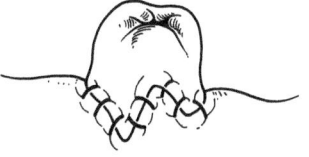

Fig.2.15. Revision of conduit stoma: use of 'Z' plasty to reduce the risk of further stenosis.

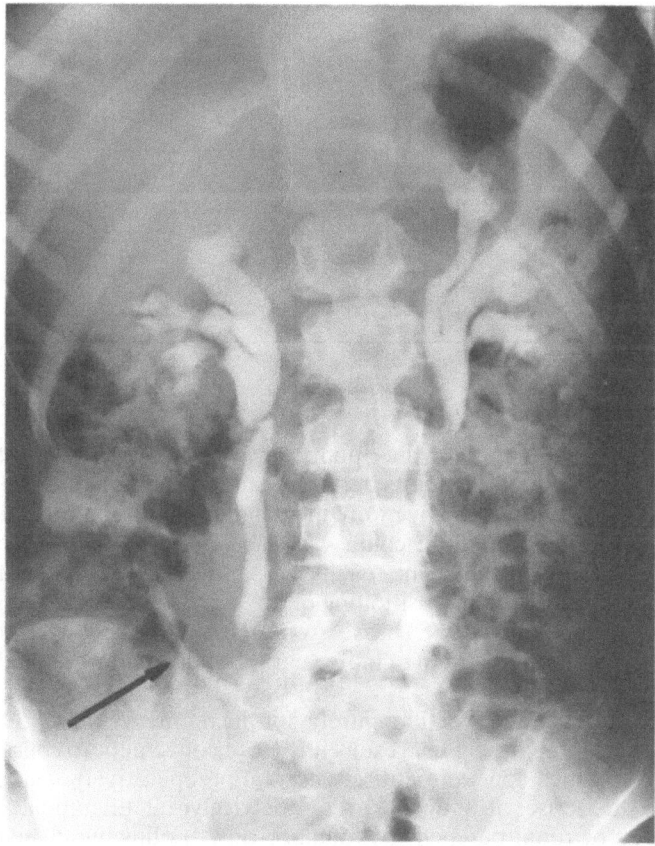

Fig.2.16. Loopogram (30-min drainage film) showing total conduit stenosis occurring 5 years post-operatively. There is free ureteric reflux but drainage is poor with narrowing of the conduit throughout its length (*arrowed*). The stoma appeared quite normal.

Refluxing Conduits

In view of the multitude of complications, it would be optimistic indeed to expect the results to be anything approaching ideal. The reported incidence of upper tract complications varies enormously, and can only partly be explained by variable length of follow-up. A summary of the findings from a selection of larger series is found in Table 2.2.

Table 2.2.   The upper renal tracts following refluxing conduits in children

Authors	No. of cases	Follow-up years	Upper tracts normal prior to diversion: Incidence of deterioration (%)	Upper tracts dilated prior to diversion		
				Improved %	Same %	Worse %
Cook et al (1958)	57	1–5	29	–	–	–
Bay and de Domenico (1972)	66	1–14	32	40	28	32
Smith (1972)	150	2–15	10	15	60	25
Middleton and Henderson (1976)	90	5–20	77	–	–	–
Stevens and Eckstein (1977)	113	1–13	9	51	32	17
Pitts and Muecke (1979)	115	0–5	6	–	–	–
		6–10	10			
		11–15	30			
		16–20	39			

During the preparation of this chapter the opportunity was taken to review the long-term results of the 131 refluxing conduits performed at the Sheffield Children's Hospital in 1960–1969. One hundred and five were indicated for neurological and 26 for non-neurological conditions. Sigmoid colon was used in 25 patients and 34 conduits were placed extra-peritoneally. The results were influenced neither by the nature of the indication nor the type or positioning of the conduit, and the series is presented as a whole. Because of death (8 cases, 5 renal), or loss to follow-up, full clinical and radiological information for ten or more years after diversion is limited to 100 cases.

Fifty eight patients underwent diversion purely for incontinence and 73 for deteriorating upper tracts. In analysing the results it is more convenient to consider individual renal units, of which 155 were entirely normal preoperatively, and 105 abnormal, usually in the sense of showing ureteropelvicalyceal dilatation, but occasionally of a degree of renal parenchymal damage only. Following diversion significant renal parenchymal damage can develop and progress even when there is no, or only minimal, upper tract dilatation (Fig. 2.17a,b), and this is taken into account when presenting the results in cases where the upper tracts had previously

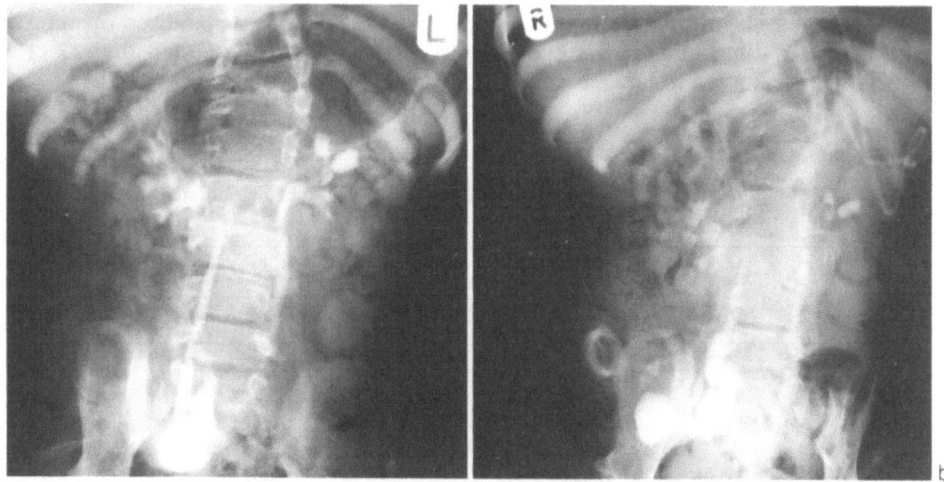

a   b

Fig. 2.17. a I.V.P. 6 years after construction of ileal conduit. There is minimal upper tract dilatation but some calyceal clubbing and renal parenchymal atrophy in the left upper pole. **b** I.V.P. 2 years later shows no further dilatation but there is now severe parenchymal damage affecting the whole of the left kidney.

been normal. Because a degree of ureteric dilatation or of parenchymal damage confined to one pole of the kidney is so common in this group after diversion, both, either alone or together, are reluctantly accepted as 'normal'. By deterioration is meant a degree of pelvicalyceal dilatation (with or without parenchymal damage) or of parenchymal damage alone affecting more than one pole of the kidney. The findings are set out in Table 2.3. Space does not allow full justice to be given to these

Table 2.3. Sheffield Children's Hospital Series 1960–1969: upper tracts normal prior to conduit diversion (n = 155)

		I.V.P.			
				Deteriorated	
Years post-diversion	Renal units available for study	Normal	Dilatation	Parenchymal damage	Total
1–2	146	110 (75%)	31 (21.5%)	5 (3.5%)	36 (25%)
5–6	132	76 (58%)	48 (36%)	8 (6%)	56 (42%)
10–12	116	53 (46%)	46 (39%)	17 (15%)	63 (54%)
15–18	50	12 (24%)	30 (60%)	8 (16%)	38 (76%)

See text for definition of findings.

figures, but it suffices to comment that in many instances renal function has been severely affected (one patient is on dialysis), and that approximately a third of the episodes of deterioration did not appear to have an obstructive basis.

In cases where upper tract deterioration predated diversion (Table 2.4), assessment of the results has been made purely in terms of ureteropelvic dilatation. Although this conceals a great deal of parenchymal damage, it does at least provide encouragement in that for many patients, conduit diversion stabilised or improved drainage of the kidneys for several years. It remains to be added that 17 (13%) patients are known to have formed stones and new cases crop up each year.

Table 2.4. Sheffield Children's Hospital Series 1960–1969: upper tracts deteriorated prior to conduit diversion (n = 105)

Years post-diversion	Renal units available for study	I.V.P.		
		Improved	No change	Worse
1–2	93	49 (52%)	36 (39%)	8 (9%)
5–6	88	45 (51%)	28 (32%)	15 (17%)
10–12	84	39 (46%)	34 (41%)	11 (13%)
15–18	36	9 (25%)	14 (42%)	12 (33%)

See text for definition of findings.

These results, and others from long-term series, prompt the conclusion that except in circumstances where it cannot be avoided, *the refluxing conduit is best regarded as an absolute procedure for children.*

Non-Refluxing Conduits

For many years Mogg (Mogg 1967; Mogg and Syme 1969) was the major, and almost the only, advocate of the anti-refluxing colonic conduit, but the indifferent results of refluxing conduits have prompted an increasing interest in this form of diversion. Further support has come from animal experiments (Richie and Skinner 1975; Kaswick et al. 1978), although it would be unwise to strictly equate the effects of reflux on the canine and the human kidney. Medium-term follow-up suggests that the results, while not perfect, represent an appreciable improvement on those obtained by the ileal conduit (Altwein et al. 1977; Althausen et al. 1978). The one series with long-term (10 years plus) follow-up (Elder et al. 1979) gives a rather different picture, with incidence of stomal stenosis (61.5%), uretero-conduit obstruction (22%), stone (16%) and upper tract deterioration (61%) rather exceeding those reported in most series of ileal conduits, although in fairness it should be noted that reflux was present in rather more than half the cases, and where this had been successfully prevented, the incidence of upper tract deterioration was much less.

On balance, the anti-refluxing colonic conduit would seem to be the preferred form of permanent diversion for children, although it may be doubted whether results in the very long long-term will prove anything like ideal.

Undiversion

The operative closure of urinary stomas never intended to be more than temporary is quite routine. What is new, and likely to increase, is reconstruction of the urinary tracts in patients who have previously undergone 'permanent' diversion. This concept was introduced by Hendren (1973) and termed 'undiversion'. At the present time it is probably fair to say that the majority of reported undiversions have been in patients who, ideally managed by current standards, would never have undergone diversion in the first place. This applies particularly in cases where the function of the bladder is normal, or can be relatively easily rendered so (e.g., posterior urethral valves). Most permanent urinary diversions in children have been performed for frank neuro-vesical dysfunction leading to incontinence or upper tract deterioration considered unmanageable by conservative means. It now seems that much more 'use' can be made of these bladders than was previously thought possible (Chap. 1), and it is quite likely that undiversion will be increasingly practised in patients with neurological disease.

Before embarking on undiversion, the surgeon must always be satisfied on two counts, firstly that the procedure will not compromise, or further compromise, existing renal function, and secondly that the patient's quality of life will be improved. In answering these questions, each case will require careful evaluation of all the relevant physical, and even psychological, factors.

Prerequisites for Undiversion

1) The renal reserve should be sufficient to cope with the scale of surgery being contemplated.

2) Any obstruction or reflux distal to the proposed reconstruction should be corrected first. Where it is intended to incorporate distal ureter in the reconstruction it may be necessary to undertake preliminary reimplantation in order to correct uretero-vesical obstruction or vesico-ureteric reflux. Such 'dry' reimplantations (i.e. with no urine passing through the uretero-vesical anastomosis) are apt to become obstructed by overgrowing bladder mucosa unless a trans-anastomotic split is left in situ for some period post-operatively. Hendren (1978b) recommends the splint be retained until the definitive undiversion, but in the author's hands, 2 weeks has proved a sufficient period.

3) The bladder must be 'safe' and usable. In patients with a normally innervated bladder this means, in practical terms, that any organic outlet obstruction has been relieved and that the bladder has adequate capacity. Capacity may be reduced either by virtue of a structural deficiency of the sphincteric mechanism, which in some instances is amenable to repair (Leadbetter 1964; Williams and Snyder 1976; Hendren 1980), or by virtue of contracture from long-standing disuse. This latter may respond to repeated distension of the bladder, or, rarely, may require some form of augmentation procedure (e.g. caecocystoplasty).

A simple means of checking continence, capacity and residual urine is to insert a suprapubic catheter through which slow filling of the bladder (50 ml/h) is conducted over a period of a week or so (Kogan and Levitt 1977).

In patients with neuro-vesical dysfunction the position is less straightforward, and the reader is referred to Chap. 1 for a discussion of the means of investigating and managing the neurogenic bladder.

4) In a few patients who have previously undergone cystectomy, or who have a bladder which is clearly unusable (e.g. severe cases of extrophy), but who retain normal, or near normal, upper renal tracts and good rectal control, consideration may be given to some form of undiversion into the colon in continuity (Chap. 3).

Indications for Undiversion

Patients with Normally Innervated Bladders

In this group it is usually clear if the bladder is capable of normal function, either *ab initio* or following reconstructive surgery. Once this has been established, undiversion is usually quite justifiable even if this involves major surgery.

Patients with Neuro-Vesical Dysfunction

Although it is now possible to secure continence in many patients with neurogenic bladder dysfunction, it must be realised that this is not continence by normal means and that most methods of management require a degree of motivation, self-discipline and skill on the part of the patient. These are not always present and, more often than not, the quality of life is better secured by persisting with an established diversion. Undiversion should only be considered when this is clearly not the case, that is:

a) Difficulty of fitting appliances due to severe spinal deformity, and where no suitable alternative stoma site exists. This is the usual indication, and is becoming increasingly common. An alternative policy in this situation is to construct a 'continent' diversion (Chap. 6).

b) Psychological problems associated with an abdominal stoma. Although sometimes a genuine indication in its own right, this may also be a manifestation of a general psychiatric disorder. A psychiatric opinion should be sought before embarking on undiversion for this indication.

c) Where continence can be simply secured via the bladder, and undiversion is technically without difficulty.

Technical Considerations

Cutaneous Ureterostomies

a) Sober and ring ureterostomies
All that is usually required is mobilisation of the stomal limb(s) to the junction with the 'main line' of the urinary tract. The limb(s) is excised at this level and the defect in the ureter or renal pelvis closed.

b) Loop ureterostomy
Following this procedure it is not uncommon to find that the distal ureter has narrowed down to almost normal size and that any vesico-ureteric reflux has resolved (Rabinowitz et al. 1977). Should reimplantation of the ureter be necessary, problems may be encountered in mobilising sufficient length, especially when the ureterostomy has been sited low. If care is taken with the blood supply, it possible to close the ureterostomy and reimplant the ureter simultaneously (Hendren 1978b). An alternative is to close the ureterostomy first and reimplant later, but this puts the kidney at some risk.

Although simple anterior closure of loop ureterostomy has been suggested (Johnston 1963) it is customary to excise the stoma and construct an oblique end-to-end ureteric anastomosis. This may be performed over an 8F or 10F T-tube with the limb brought out distal to the anastomosis. It is removed some 10 days postoperatively. With high loop ureterostomies it is sometimes preferable to excise the proximal limb and anastomose the distal limb directly to the renal pelvis (Johnston and Kulatilake 1972).

c) End ureterostomy

Provided that the ureter was not shortened at the original procedure, there is not usually any difficulty in mobilising sufficient length for reimplantation into the bladder by whichever technique is preferred. If there is insufficient length, one of the techniques referred to in the following section will be needed.

Conduit Diversions

As a matter of general principle it is preferable to undivert without incorporating an intestinal segment. Not only is there a general impression that renal function is better preserved in this way, but in patients with neuro-vesical dysfunction which, it is intended, should be managed with a catheter (indwelling or intermittent), intestinal mucus may cause considerable problems with blockage.

Each case requires thorough preoperative radiological studies to determine the length of ureters proximally, the length of any distal ureteric stumps, and the length and function of the conduit. To accomplish undiversion without incorporating an intestinal segment may require considerable ingenuity, and among the possibilities which may be considered, alone or in combination, are the use of distal ureteric stump(s), transureteroureterostomy, psoas bladder hitch, Boari bladder flaps, extensive renal mobilisation or even renal auto-transplantation (Hendren 1978a).

On occasion the length of available ureter(s) is such that an intestinal segment must be used, either to bridge a gap between proximal and distal ureters, or to be implanted directly into the bladder. The bowel used may be either the original conduit if its function and length are satisfactory, or a new segment of intestine if they are not. It is always tempting, and often quite easy, to mobilise the conduit and anastomose the distal everted spout to the dome of the bladder. This temptation is best resisted. Experience indicates that this manoeuvre may be followed by massive reflux leading to deteriorating renal function (Hendren 1978a). If intestinal segments are to be used in children they should be tailored along their anti-mesenteric border, and, if they are to be implanted into the bladder, this should be via a long sub-mucosal tunnel.

Brendler and Stephenson (1981) in a recent review of urinary diversion and undiversion in children, emphasise that whilst the early results of undiversion have been encouraging, it is essential to have a vigilance in the long-term follow-up to try and avoid some of the complications experienced with surface diversions.

References

Allen T (1980) Vesicostomy for the temporary diversion of the urine in small children. J Urol 123: 929–931

Althausen AF, Hagen-Cook K, Hendren WH (1978) Non-refluxing colon conduit: Experience with 70 cases. J Urol 120: 35–39

Altwein JE, Jonas U, Hohenfellner R (1977) Long-term follow-up of children with colon conduit urinary diversion and ureterosigmoidostomy. J Urol 118: 832–836

Babcock JRJr, Schkolnik A, Cook WA (1979) Ultrasound-guided percutaneous nephrostomy in the pediatric patient. J Urol 121: 327–329

Barnhouse DH (1972) Prune belly syndrome. Br J Urol 44: 356–360

Bell TE, Hoodin AO, Evans AT (1968) Tubeless cystostomy in children. J Urol 100: 459–461

Bergman B, Nilson AE, Pettersson A, Sundin T (1977) Back-flow from urine collecting devices into the ileal conduit. Br J Urol 49: 503–507

Bishop RF, Smith ED, Gracey M (1971) Bacterial flora of urine from ileal conduit. J Urol 105: 452–455

Blocksum BW (1957) Bladder pouch for prolonged tubless cystostomy. J Urol 78: 398–401

Bloom DA, Turner WR, Skinner DG (1981) Urological Stomas. Modern Techniques in Surgery. Urol Surg

Brendler CB, Stephenson TP (1981) Urinary diversion and undiversion in children. J Urol 125: 457–462

Bricker EM (1950) Bladder substitution after pelvic exenteration. Surg Clin North Am 30: 1511–1521

Bruce RR, Gonzales ET (1980) Cutaneous vesicostomy: A useful form of temporary diversion in children. J Urol 123: 927–928

Campbell DP, Swenson O (1972) Wound dehiscence in infants and children. J Pediatr Surg 7: 123–126

Castro JE, Ram MD (1970) Electrolyte imbalance following ileal urinary diversion. Br J Urol 42: 29–32

Castro JE, Mustapha N, Mee AD, Shackman R (1975) Ileal urinary diversions in patients with renal transplants. Br J Urol 47: 603–606

Cook RCM, Lister J, Zachary RB (1968) Operative management of the neurogenic bladder in children: Diversion through intestinal conduits. Surgery 63: 825–831

David FRD (1976) A new surgical procedure for revision of ileal conduit stoma in children. J Urol 115: 188–190

Douglas LL (1979) Uretero-ileal anastomosis in conduit diversion. Urology 13: 78–80

Dunn M, Roberts JBM, Smith PJB, Slade N (1979) The long-term results of ileal conduit diversion in children. Br J Urol 51: 458–461

Eckstein HB, Kapila L (1970) Cutaneous ureterostomy. Br J Urol 42: 306–315

Elder DD, Moisey CU, Rees RWM (1979) A long-term follow-up of the colonic conduit operation in children. Br J Urol 51: 462–465

Emery JL, Gill GW (1974) A classification and quantitative histological study of abnormal ureters in children. Br J Urol 46: 69–79

Ezell WW, Carlson HE (1970) A realistic look at extrophy of the bladder. Br J Urol 42: 197–202

Firlit CF, Merkel FK (1977) The application of ileal conduits in pediatric renal transplantation. J Urol 118: 647–650

Gornall P, Mann JR, Corkery JJ (1979) Recent experience in the treatment of rhabdomyosarcoma. J Pediatr Surg 14: 38–40

Hanna MK, Jeffs RD, Sturgess JM, Barkin M (1977a) Ureteral structure and ultrastructure. Part III. The congenitally dilated ureter (megaureter). J Urol 117: 24–27

Hanna MK, Jeffs RD, Sturgess JM, Barkin M (1977b) Ureteral structure and ultrastructure. Part IV. The dilated ureter, clinicopathological correlation. J Urol 117: 28–33

Hendren WH (1972) Restoration of function in severely decompensated ureters. In: Johnston JH, Scholtmeijer RJ (eds) Problems in paediatric urology. Excerpta Medica, Amsterdam, pp 1–56

Hendren WH (1973) Reconstruction of previously diverted urinary tracts in children. J Ped Surg 8: 135–150

Hendren WH (1976) Extrophy of the bladder — an alternative approach. J Urol 115: 195–202

Hendren WH (1978a) Some alternatives to urinary diversion in children. J Urol 119: 652–660

Hendren WH (1978b) Complications of ureterostomy. J Urol 120: 269–281

Hendren WH (1980) Urogenital sinus and anorectal malformations: Experience with 22 cases. J Pediatr Surg 15: 628–641

Itatani H, Sonoda T (1978) New technique of antireflux ureteroileal anastomosis and its clinical experiences. J Urol 119: 735–739

Johnston JH (1963) Temporary cutaneous ureterostomy in management of advanced congenital obstructions. Arch Dis Child 38: 161–166

Johnston JH (1974) Pyelo-colonic diversion in children. Br J Urol 46: 169–172

Johnston JH, Farkas A (1975) The congenital refluxing megaureter: Experiences with surgical reconstruction. Br J Urol 47: 153–159

Johnston JH, Kulatilake AE (1971) The sequelae of posterior urethral valves. Br J Urol 43: 743–748

Johnston JH, Kulatilake AE (1972) Posterior urethral valves. In: Johnston JH, Scholtmeijer RJ (eds) Problems in paediatric urology. Excerpta Medica, Amsterdam, pp 161–179

Kafetsioulis A, Swinney J (1968) Urinary diversion by ileal conduit. Br J Urol 40: 1–11

Kafetsioulis A, Swinney J (1970) A study of the function of ileal conduits. Br J Urol 42: 33–36

Kaswick JA, Gottesman JE, Walsman J, Skinner DF (1978) Antirefluxing colon conduits for diversion of dilated upper urinary tracts. J Pediatr Surg 13: 532–533

Kogan SJ, Levitt SB (1977) Bladder evaluation in pediatric patients before undiversion in previously diverted urinary tracts. J Urol 118: 443–446

Lapides J, Ajemian EP, Lichtwardt A (1960) Cutaneous vesicostomy. J Urol 84: 609–614

Leadbetter GW (1964) Surgical correction of total urinary incontinence. J Urol 91: 261–266

Leadbetter GW, Clarke BG (1954) Five years experience with uretero-enterostomy by the 'combined' technique. J Urol 73: 67–82

Lister J, Cook RCM, Zachary RB (1968) Operative management of neurogenic bladder dysfunction in children: Ureterostomy. Arch Dis Child 43: 672–678

Lome LG, Howat JM, Williams DI (1972) The temporarily defunctionalized bladder in children. J Urol 107: 469–472

Magnus RV (1977) Pressure studies and dynamics of ileal conduits in children. J Urol 118: 405–407

Malpas JS, Freeman JE, Paxton A, Walker Smith J, Stansfeld AG, Woods CBS (1976) Radiotherapy and adjuvant combination chemotherapy for childhood rhabdomyosarcoma. Br Med J i: 247–249

Mathisen W (1953) A new method for ureterointestinal anastomosis. Surg Gynecol Obstet 96: 255–258

McEwan AB, Clark P (1973) The stoma of the ileal conduit. Br J Urol 45: 600–605

Middleton AW, Hendren WH (1976) Ileal conduits in children at the Massachusetts General Hospital from 1955 to 1970. J Urol 115: 591–595

Mitchell ME, Yoder IC, Pfister RC, Daly J, Althausen A (1977) Ileal loop stenosis: A late complication of urinary diversion. J Urol 118: 957–961

Mogg RA (1967) Urinary diversion using the colonic conduit. Br J Urol 39: 687–692

Mogg RA (1974) The single ectopic ureter. Br J Urol 46: 3–10

Mogg RA, Syme RRA (1969) The results of urinary diversion using the colonic conduit. Br J Urol 41: 434–447

Nash DFE (1956) Ileal loop bladder in congenital spinal palsy. Br J Urol 28: 387–393

Neifield JP, Maurer HM, Godwin, D, Berg JW, Salzberg AM (1979) Prognostic variables in rhabdomyosarcoma before and after multimodal therapy. J Pediatr Surg 14, 699–703

O'Reilly PH, Testa HJ, Lawson RS, Farrar DJ, Charlton Edwards E (1978) Diuresis renography in equivocal urinary tract obstruction. Br J Urol 50: 76–80

Pekarovič E, Robinson A, Lister J, Zachary RB (1968) Pressure variations in intestinal loops used for urinary diversion. Dev Med Child Neurol [Suppl] 16: 87–92

Philp N, Richwood AMK (1981) Management of vesico-ureteric reflux in the congenital neuropathic bladder. Br J Urol 00: 00–00

Pitts WRJr, Muecke EC (1979) A 20-year experience with ileal conduits: The fate of the kidneys. J Urol 122: 154–157

Poor P, Kursh ED, Persky L (1975) The add-on ileal loop. J Urol 114: 281–284

Rabinowitz R, Barkin M. Schillinger JF, Jeffs RD, Cook GT (1977) Surgical management of the massively dilated ureter in children. II. Management by primary reconstruction. J Urol 118: 436–439

Rabinowitz R, Barkin M, Schillinger JF, Jeffs RD, Cook GT (1972a) Surgical management of massive neurogenic hydronephrosis. J Urol 122: 64–65

Rabinowitz R, Barkin M, Schillinger JF, Jeffs RD, Cook GT (1979b) Upper tract management when posterior urethral valve ablation is insufficient. J Urol 122: 370–372

Ray P, de Dominico I (1972) Intestinal conduit urinary diversion in children. Br J Urol 44: 345–350

Richie JP, Skinner DG (1975) Urinary diversion: The physiological rationale for non-refluxing colonic conduits. Br J Urol 47: 269–275

Rickwood AMK (1978) Urinary tract calculi in childhood, a 10 year survey. Problemy Chirurgii Dzieciecej 5: 32–41

Rickwood AMK, Hemalatha V, Brooman P (1979) Closure of colostomy in infants and children. Br J Surg 66: 273–279

Sadlowski RW, Belman AB, Filmer RB, Smey P, King LR (1978) Follow up of cutaneous ureterostomy in children. J Urol 119: 116–119

Sadlowski RW, Finney RP, Branch WT, Rosenthal NS, Sharpe JR (1979) New technique for percutaneous nephrostomy under ultrasound guidance. J Urol 121: 559–561

Scott JES (1973) Urinary diversion in children. Arch Dis Child 48: 199–206

Smith ED (1965) Spina bifida and the total care of myelomeningocoele. Thomas, Springfield, Illinois

Smith ED (1972) Follow-up studies of 150 ileal conduits in children. J Pediatr Surg 7: 1–10

Snyder HM, Harrison NW, Whitfield HN, Williams DI (1976) Urodynamics in the prune belly syndrome. Br J Urol 48: 663–670

Sober I (1972) Pelvioureterostomy-en-Y. J Urol 107: 473–475

Stevens PS, Eckstein HB (1975) The management of pyocystis following ileal conduit urinary diversion in children. Br J Urol 47: 631–633

Stevens PS, Eckstein HB (1977) Ileal conduit urinary diversion in children. Br J Urol 49: 379–383

Stewart WW, Cass AS, Matsen JM (1979) Bacteriuria with intestinal loop urinary diversion in children. J Urol 122: 528–531

Sukarochana K, Sicker WK (1978) Vesicointestinal fistula revisited. J Pediatr Surg 13: 713–718

Sweitzer SJ, Kelalis PP (1978) Cutaneous transureteroureterostomy as a form of diversion in children with a compromised urinary tract. J Urol 120: 589–591

Turner-Warwick RT, Ashken MH (1967) The functional results of partial, subtotal and total cystoplasty with special reference to ureterocaecocystoplasty, selective sphincterotomy and cystocystoplasty. Br J Urol 39: 3–12

Wallace DM (1970) Uretero-ileostomy. Br J Urol 42: 529–534

Whitaker RH (1973) Methods of assessing obstruction in dilated ureters. Br J Urol 45: 15–22

Whitaker RH (1979) An evaluation of 170 diagnostic pressure flow studies of the upper urinary tract. J Urol 121: 602–604

Whitfield HN, Harrison NW, Sherwood T, Williams DI (1976) Upper urinary tract obstruction: Pressure/flow studies in children. Br J Urol 48: 427–430

Whitfield HN, Britton KE, Hendry WF, Nimmon CC, Wickham JEA (1978) The distinction between obstructive uropathy and nephropathy by radioisotope transit times. Br J Urol 50: 433–436

Williams DI (1972) Reconstructive surgery for extrophy of the bladder. In: Johnston JH, Scholtmeijer RJ (eds) Problems in paediatric urology. Excerpta Medica, Amsterdam, pp 79–90

Williams DI, Bloomberg S (1976) Urogenital sinus in the female child. J Pediatr Surg 11: 51–56

Williams DI, Cromie WJ (1975) Ring ureterostomy. Br J Urol 47: 789–792

Williams DI, Hulme-Moir I (1970) Primary obstructive megaureter. Br J Urol 42: 140–149

Williams DI, Keeton JE (1973) Further progress with reconstruction of the extrophied bladder. Br J Surg 60: 203–207

Williams DI, Lightwood RG (1972) Bilateral single ectopic ureters. Br J Urol 44: 267–273

Williams DI, Parker RM (1974) The role of surgery in the prune belly syndrome. In: Johnston JH, Goodwin WE (eds) Reviews in paediatric urology. Excerpta Medica, Amsterdam

Williams DI, Rabinovitch HH (1967) Cutaneous ureterostomy for the grossly dilated ureter of childhood. Br J Urol 39: 696–699

Williams DI, Snyder H (1976) Anterior detrusor tube repair for urinary incontinence in children. Br J Urol 48: 671–674

Williams DI, Whitaker RH, Barratt TM, Keeton JE (1973) Urethral valves. Br J Urol 45: 200–210

Woodhouse CRJ, Kellett MJ, Williams DI (1979) Minimal surgical interference in the prune belly syndrome. Br J Urol 51: 475–480

Woodburn ME (1973) Social implications of spina bifida — a study in S E Scotland. Scottish Spina Bifida Association, Eastern Branch, Edinburgh

Chapter 3

Ureterosigmoidostomy in Children

Michael Marberger and Eberhard Straub

In 1973, Megalli and Lattimer summed up 25 years experience with uretero-sigmoidostomy in children: '. . . all patients had some degree of acidosis, hyperchloremia and electrolyte disturbance. In 26 of the 30 there was some degree of upper tract deterioration on one or both sides with recurrent pyelonephritis. Fifteen patients underwent nephrectomy and 13 patients had stone formation at various levels of the urinary tract. There were 3 cases of symptomatic polyps at a ureteral orifice requiring removal. Ten patients subsequently underwent a different type of diversion. Three patients have died.'

These lines reflect the general dismay with the poor late results of uretero-sigmoidostomy, which led to almost complete abandonment of the technique in favour of conduit diversion. Today, however, there is a growing disillusion in respect to the long-term results of ileal (Elder et al. 1979; Schwartz et al. 1976; Schwartz and Jeffs 1975) and colonic (Dunn et al. 1979; Marberger et al. to be published) conduits, too, renewing interest in ureterosigmoidostomy. Bakker and Cornil (1974), Zincke and Segura (1975), Spence et al. (1975) and Goodwin and Scardino (1977) showed that restriction of ureterosigmoidostomy to children with a normal upper urinary tract and colon and a scrutinous follow-up considerably ameliorated the results as compared to the figures quoted above. Improvements in operative techniques, in particular in prevention of colo-ureteric reflux and stenosis (Mathisen 1953; Goodwin and Scardino 1977; Hohenfellner 1977) and efficient management of metabolic disorders (Heidler et al. 1979) eliminate many of the problems responsible for ureterosigmoidostomy's earlier disrepute. In view of the enormous advantage of avoiding a stoma, ureterosigmoidostomy must therefore today again be considered for urinary diversion in a selected group of children.

Prerequisites for Success

Correct Patient Selection

The crucial point of ureterosigmoidostomy arises from the diversion of sterile urine into the contaminated intestinal tract. Upper urinary tract infection is prevented if the uretero-intestinal anastomosis is neither obstructive nor refluxing. Even with an optimum technique, this can only be achieved with healthy tissue. Patients with scarred or dilated ureters or a sigmoid damaged by inflammation, irradiation or previous surgery must therefore be excluded from the procedure. In a detailed follow-up study of ureterosigmoidostomy in adults, 55% of the patients in whom these criteria were ignored suffered complications, compared to a morbidity rate of 22% in patients selected correctly. Colo-ureteric reflux was twice as common in ureters dilated preoperatively even if the ureters were tailored (Marberger et al. to be published). For the same reason, ureterosigmoidostomy cannot be followed by postoperative irradiation of the pelvic region.

With normal renal function, metabolic imbalances resulting from chloride re-absorption and chronic alkali and potassium losses can be managed satisfactorily by oral substitution; some children may not even require life-long treatment. With deteriorating renal function from pyelonephritis or obstruction, the self-regulatory compensating mechanisms rapidly break down, giving way to severe derangements of acid-base and electrolyte metabolism (Pinck et al. 1975; Heidler et al. 1979). In a follow-up series of 67 adults with ureterosigmoidostomy, 2 of 4 patients submitted to the procedure in spite of radiological signs of pyelonephritis experienced severe metabolic complications; hyperchloraemic acidosis requiring hospitalisation was only observed in cases with pyelonephritis and/or ureteral dilatation (Heidler et al. 1979). A normal upper urinary tract and colon as demonstrated on an excretory urogram and barium enema are therefore mandatory.

With social rehabilitation of the ureterosigmoidostomy patient being based on complete anal continence of urine, an intact anal sphincter mechanism is essential. Where this cannot be reliably met, such as in children with neurogenic bladder dysfunction or abnormalities of the rectum, the procedure is contraindicated. The ability to retain an enema of 150–250 ml lukewarm saline usually guarantees anal continence. The decision may become difficult in very young children with exstrophy, in whom associated anal dysfunction is common and complete control of the anal sphincter often not acquired before the twelfth year of age. Elaborate intrarectal pressure studies or electromyography of the anal sphincter muscle may provide some help; in the authors' experience, digital palpation of the sphincter has proven almost as reliable. With a good sphincter tonus, anal continence of urine can be expected. Nevertheless, children with a history of rectal prolapse should be excluded from ureterosigmoidostomy.

Non-Refluxing Implantation Technique

The impact of ureterosigmoidostomy on the upper urinary tract is directly related to the success with which a neat mucosa-to-mucosa anastomosis with an anti-reflux mechanism is achieved (Clarke and Leadbetter 1955). Two methods are most commonly used to obtain this objective: the formation of an intraluminal nipple (Mathisen 1953) or an elliptical anastomosis with a submucosal tunnel (Goodwin et al. 1953; Clarke and Leadbetter 1955; Hohenfellner 1977). The authors exclusively employ the latter principle in the Hohenfellner modification (1977) of Goodwin's transcolonic method (Goodwin et al. 1953).

The surgical technique has been reported elsewhere in detail (Hohenfellner 1977); a teaching film is available (Hohenfellner and Marberger 1980). In short, the ureters are transected as close as possible to the bladder and mobilised carefully preserving their blood supply. The lower sigmoid is opened along a taenia coli and the

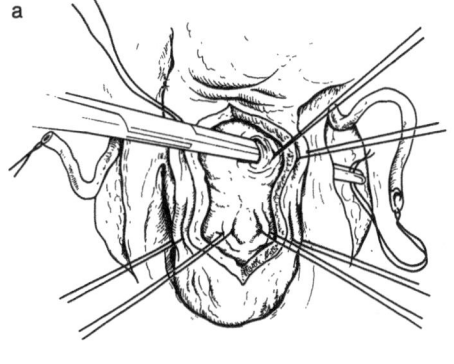

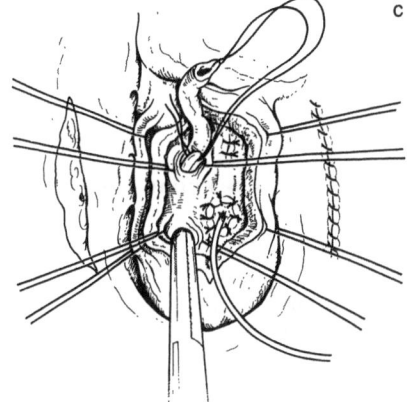

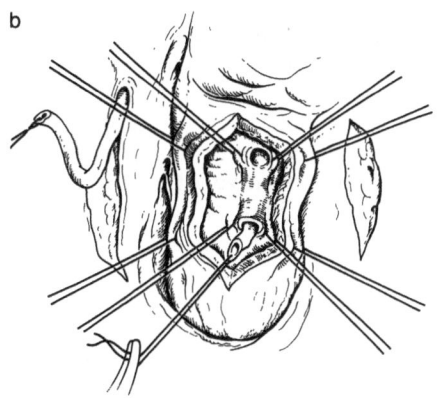

Fig. 3.1. Transcolonic ureterosigmoidostomy.
a A haemostat is advanced through a buttonhole
in the posterior sigmoid wall, tunnelling precisely
below the visceral peritoneum. The stay suture
of the mobilised left ureter is grasped. **b** The
ureter is pulled into the intestinal lumen and on
through a submucosal tunnel formed between
the four stay sutures. **c** With the mucosa-to-
mucosa anastomosis of the left ureter completed
and splinted, the right ureter is implanted with
an identical technique. From Hohenfellner
(1977), with permission.

implantation site marked with stay sutures on the inner posterior sigmoid wall. A
buttonhole of mucosa and musculature is excised and a straight haemostat advanced
laterally to one of the ureters in a plane just below the peritoneal cover of the
mesosigmoid (Fig. 3.1a). By spreading of the jaws of the haemostat a tunnel is formed
along which the ureter is brought into the intestinal lumen. The stay sutures are then
tautened to flatten the mucosa so that a submucosal tunnel 3–4 cm in length can be
modelled in the posterior sigmoid wall, very much as in ureteroneocystostomy (Fig.
3.1b). The ureter is threaded through the tunnel, spatulated and anastomosed
precisely to the intestinal mucosa with 5–0 chromic catgut sutures. The most distal
suture also grasps musculature to anchor the anastomosis. The contralateral ureter is
implanted in an identical manner in a slightly more lateral and proximal or distal
position (Fig. 3.1c). Both ureters are splinted with graduated polyvinyl tubes, which
are led out through the rectum with the help of a rectal tube. The tube is reinserted at
the end of the procedure.

With this technique, intestinal peristalsis remains undisturbed and the ureters
course freely through the mesosigmoid being attached to the bowels at the site of the
anastomosis only. With a very mobile sigmoid, however, the anastomosis may come
under tension by the weight of the sigmoid, especially on the right side and with a
rather high implantation (Walz and Alken 1980). If this seems possible, it is advisable
to reduce sigmoid mobility slightly by tacking the mesosigmoid to the promontory on

each side with two anchoring sutures. All difficult phases of the anastomoses are performed under direct vision and reflux is prevented (Marberger et al. to be published).

Postoperative Follow-up

A child may only be subjected to ureterosigmoidostomy if life-long urological surveillance seems warranted. Follow-up examinations are performed routinely after 3 months, 6 months, 12 months and thereafter at yearly intervals. Besides the physical check-up this includes exact evaluation of the electrolyte and acid-base metabolism, a scout film of the abdomen and an excretory urogram. To reduce radiation exposure, the latter is reduced to one film 30 min after the injection of contrast; as the amount of contrast/kg body weight administered remains the same, the different urograms are comparable. With signs of renal deterioration, renal function should be quantified by split radioisotope clearance studies. Starting 5 years post-operatively, stools should be checked for blood every 4 months, and a sigmoidoscopy or barium enema performed at 5-year intervals. Naturally, the pattern of follow-up is intensified with any symptoms indicative of the urinary tract or colon, during pregnancies, or with any pathological findings.

Metabolic Substitution Therapy

The continuous contact of urine with the rectal mucosa results in chronic resorption of urea and Cl^-. In the presence of urease-producing bacteria, urea is split to ammonium with the effect of a continuous ammonium chloride influx into the blood (Koff 1975). In addition, potassium is lost in excess by secretion from the colonic mucosa and renal loss due to the increased osmotic diuresis (Chisolm 1977). With normal renal function, an increased renal reabsorption of HCO_3^- and K^+ may in part prevent severe metabolic imbalances. With deteriorating renal compensatory mechanisms due to pyelonephritis, obstruction or dehydration, hyperchloraemic hypokalaemic acidosis with life-threatening sequelae rapidly develops (Heidler et al. 1975).

Metabolic problems are reliably prevented if children with abnormal renal function are excluded from ureterosigmoidostomy and if the potassium and alkali losses are replaced by long-term oral supplementation. The authors routinely administer calcium-sodium-citrate or calcium-magnesium-citrate, which are commercially available as well-palatable granules (*Acetolyt®, Uralyt-U®, Madaus*, FRG). The dosage is adjusted individually according to regular blood-gas and serum electrolyte analyses and normally ranges from 70–140 mg/kg body weight. More sophisticated methods of evaluating potassium depletion, like the determination of whole-body-potassium or of intracellular electrolyte values provide no substantial improvement of metabolic surveillance (Boddy et al. 1975; Heidler et al. 1975). The children are, however, urged to drink plenty of fluid and to empty their rectum every 3–4 h during daytime and at least once at night. In addition, they are maintained on low-dose prophylactic chemotherapy over at least 6 months postoperatively.

As incipient hyperchloraemic acidosis rarely causes specific symptoms the patients frequently find it difficult to understand the need for long-term metabolic surveillance and treatment. Ureterosigmoidostomy is therefore only advisable in patients ready to accept long-term follow-up. Should acute pyelonephritis occur, the metabolic supervision and substitution therapy should be intensified (Heidler et al. 1979).

Conversion to Colonic Conduit

In case of renal deterioration, the ureterosigmoidostomy must rapidly be converted to a low-pressure conduit-type diversion to prevent further loss of renal parenchyma. The authors consider a non-refluxing colonic conduit the optimum alternative; with very short ureters, the colonic segment may be modelled from the transverse colon (Alken et al. 1978; Marberger et al. to be published). The original uretero-intestinal anastomoses have to be excised completely to prevent later colonic malignancies at the implantation site (Pierce et al. 1978; Spence et al. 1978). It is extremely important that the patients, or with children, the parents, be made aware of this possibility and fully agree to it even before the ureterosigmoidostomy is performed. Once patients have experienced the ureterosigmoidostomy and the perfect social rehabilitation obtained therewith, it becomes difficult to convince them of the need of a stoma after renal complications. The conversion of a ureterosigmoidostomy to a rectal bladder by diverting faeces with a colostomy results in severe psychological problems in children, and should be avoided.

Indication

With respect to the prerequisites cited above, ureterosigmoidostomy must be restricted to a small group of children with defects limited to the lower urinary tract. The most important clinical entity is bladder exstrophy. Although at the present time enthusiasm for functional closure is reviving, only a few patients with large elastic bladders and without polypoid thickening of the mucosa will profit substantially from a staged reconstructive approach (Arap et al. 1980); most cases ultimately require urinary diversion. Untreated exstrophy almost always presents with a normal upper urinary tract (Spence et al. 1975), and children with anal sphincter incompetence can usually be readily identified. Primary diversion with a ureterosigmoidostomy and excision of the bladder plate will offer excellent social rehabilitation for the majority of these children and some series report very encouraging late results well worth comparing with other approaches in management (Bakker and Cornill 1974; Spence et al. 1975; Bettex 1977). Likewise, children with incontinence from total epispadias or traumatic lesions of the urethra, in whom reconstruction failed, may occasionally require ureterosigmoidostomy. The rare cases of pelvic malignancies needing cystectomy may only be diverted by ureterosigmoidostomy if adjuvant irradiation can definitely be excluded from therapy. At least for rhabdomyosarcoma, this at present does not appear to be justified.

Postoperative Complications

In general, the procedure is well tolerated. To reduce postoperative ileus, the children are maintained on a standardised intravenous hyperalimentation therapy and bowel distention is prevented with a nasogastric tube. The ureteral splints are removed sequentially around the tenth postoperative day, and the rectal tube the day thereafter. Occasionally this may result in a short spell of fever, which, however, usually subsides within hours under forced fluid intake. The antibiotic coverage begins with a potent agent at the time of surgery. Oral substitution of alkali and potassium losses is commenced at the time the child begins to retain urine in the rectum.

A detailed report of the postoperative course of 39 children and adolescents subjected to ureterosigmoidostomy was presented elsewhere (Marberger et al. to be published). Two children required surgery because of bowel obstruction — precise closure of all peritoneal defects acting as potential small bowel 'traps' appears advisable. A uretero-cutaneous fistula closed spontaneously after temporary nephrostomy drainage. Major wound dehiscence occurred twice; both children had bladder exstrophy, simultaneous excision of the bladder and reconstruction of the abdominal wall without a pelvic osteotomy. As there were no other serious surgical complications in this series, the overall complication rate was calculated at 13%, which seems to be an acceptable figure when comparing it to the morbidity of alternative techniques.

The excretory urogram is repeated prior to hospital discharge. In general the ureters appear slightly distended due to oedema at the implantation site, but this should have resolved by the time of the next radiological control 3 months later. Among the six children operated on at the Mainz University Hospital since the report mentioned above, two showed continuing obstruction proximal to the anastomosis from an acute stenosis. The implantation technique had been slightly varied in these in an attempt to anchor the ureters to the mesosigmoid. This method was subsequently abandoned and has not been used since. Both ureters were successfully reimplanted by an identical technique slightly proximal to the original implantation site some weeks later, after temporary nephrostomy drainage.

Late Results and Complications

For an update review of the long-term results, 16 children were investigated at a recall examination. All had had their ureterosigmoidostomy performed at the University of Mainz Medical School 1968–1975, a time for which all pertinent patient records and roentgenograms were still available and during which the surgical technique and postoperative management remained unchanged. The follow-up thus obtained ranged from 12.5 to 5.1 years with a mean of 9.7 years. Urinary diversion was exclusively performed because of exstrophy or severe epispadias. The age at the time of operation varied from 3 months to 14 years (mean 4.5 years). In four children a previous attempt at functional reconstruction of bladder exstrophy had failed, leaving the children incontinent. In one patient a Boyce-Vest urinary diversion was converted to ureterosigmoidostomy because of colostomy problems and severe vesicoureteric reflux (Fig. 3.2a–d). With one exception, these patients represent all children subjected to ureterosigmoidostomy during this period. The only patient not available for a recall examination had a ureterosigmoidostomy and simultaneous cystectomy performed for a rhabdomyosarcoma 8 years ago. He is under the care of a pediatric oncology centre and is reported to be without complaints, but had to be admitted to hospital treatment twice in the past because of severe metabolic acidosis.

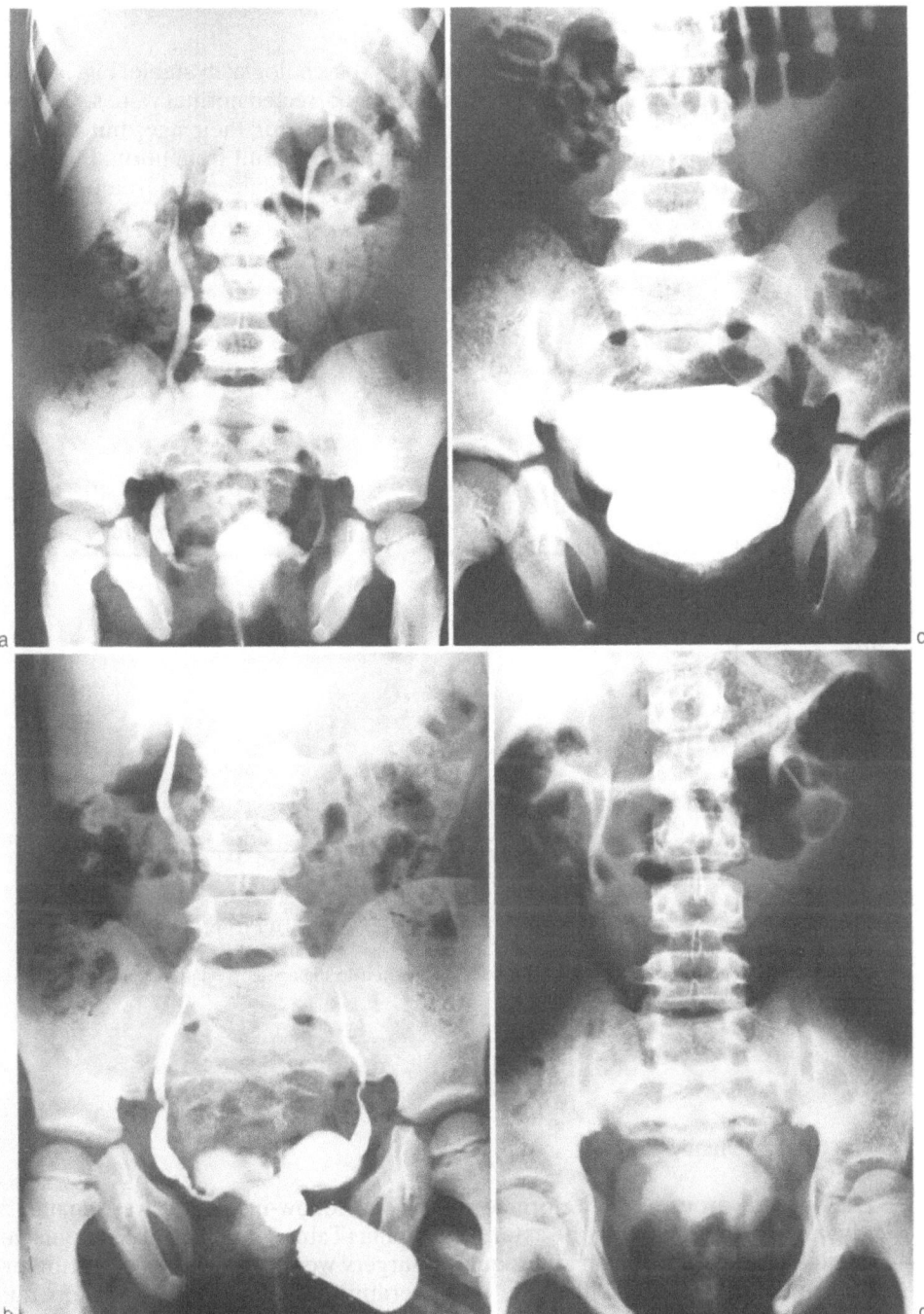

Fig.3.2. Boy, 3 years after vesicorectal anastomosis and colostomy (Boyce-Vest procedure) because of bladder exstrophy. Excretory urogram (**a**) and cystogram (**b**)—bilateral vesico-ureteric reflux. Conversion to ureterosigmoidostomy, asymptomatic since liquid-dye enema (**c**) showing no colo-ureteral reflux 2 years after ureterosigmoidostomy, and excretory urogram (**d**) 9 years after ureterosigmoidostomy. Radiograms of Figs 3.2 and 3.4 courtesy of Dr. I. Greinacher, Pediatric Radiology, University of Mainz Medical School.

Growth

All children appeared healthy and physically and psychologically stable. Fig. 3.3 gives
the body length and weight correlated to the age-corrected normal values. Only two
children were significantly below the normal length for their age, but both had
extremely small parents so that the length deficit may result from normal variation.
Otherwise there were no signs indicative of retarded or abnormal development.

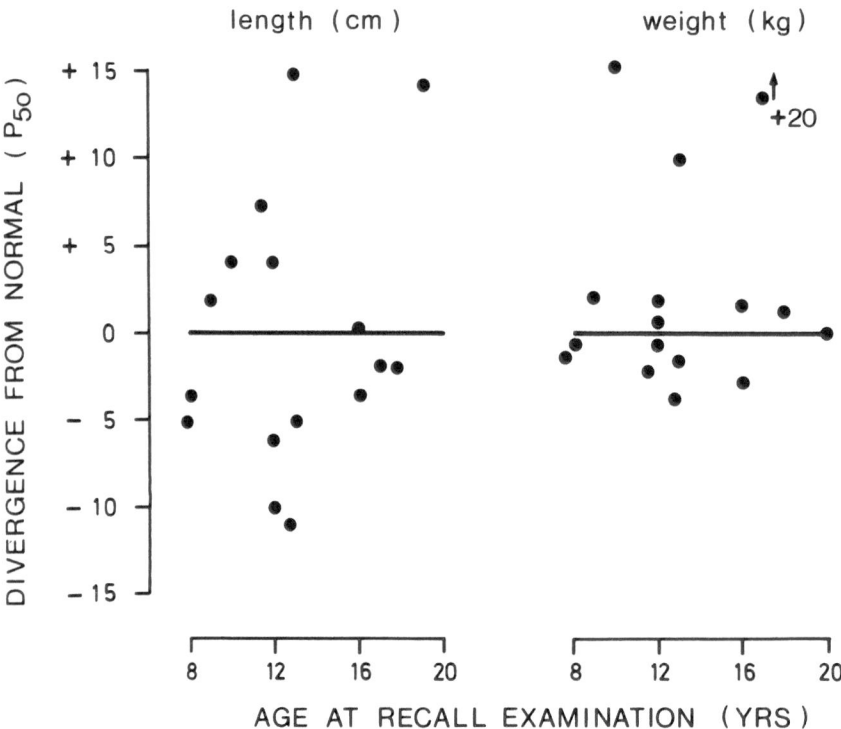

Fig.3.3. Length and body weight of 16 patients correlated to the age-corrected normal mean 9.7 years
after ureterosigmoidostomy in childhood.

The Upper Urinary Tract

The surgical procedures performed during the follow-up period were mainly reconstructive operations on the external genitalia (Table 3.1). The only complications
related to urinary diversion and requiring surgery were two stenoses of the ureter at
the implantation site. Neither the intraoperative technique nor the postoperative
course offered an explanation for the problems which were observed 16 and 18
months postoperatively. Both stenoses developed insidiously without symptoms;
they were discovered on routine intravenous urograms after previous urograms had
been normal. As with the two cases of acute ureteric obstruction the situations were
managed successfully by temporary nephrostomy drainage and subsequent reim-
planatation of the ureter.

Table 3.1. Surgical procedures performed in 16 children following ureterosigmoidostomy (mean follow-up 9.7 years).

Closure of wound dehiscence (postoperative complications)	1
Inguinal herniotomy	3
Reconstruction of penis	6
Orchidopexy	1
Vaginoplasty	2
Incision of scrotal abscess	1
Ureteral reimplantation (late stenosis)	2

All children had an intravenous urogram at the time of their late recall examination. One kidney contained a small calyceal calculus which had not caused symptoms. Two kidneys showed pyelonephritic scarring; a comparison with the preoperative films revealed that some calyceal deformity had already been present in both kidneys preoperatively, but that it had increased during the follow-up period (Fig. 3.4a–d). Both patients had been diverted after unsuccessful reconstructive attempts. Although the children had not experienced symptoms indicative of acute pyelonephritis during follow-up, their urograms demonstrate the potential hazards of primary reconstruction of bladder exstrophy. All other kidneys were normal.

In general, the urine drained promptly and without obstruction into the sigmoid (Figs. 3.3 and 3.4). One patient showed bilateral, and two unilateral ureteric dilatation which was always moderate and limited to the distal half of the ureter. The children had been asymptomatic and had not received any specific therapy. The four ureters which had been reimplanted because of stenoses were now slender and unobstructed. A contrast-dye enema was not performed at the recall examination, but ten of the 16 children had had this investigation done at an earlier time. Colo-ureteric reflux was never noticed (Figs. 3.2 and 3.4). Air was never observed in the urinary tract.

No patient lost a kidney, and renal function remained uniformly stable. Figure 3.5 gives the serum creatinine and blood urea values. Whereas the former were always normal, blood urea levels were usually elevated due to an increased reabsorption of urea via the rectal mucosa — a common finding in ureterosigmoidostomy (Chisolm 1977). Using a formula developed by Schwartz et al. 1976, the glomerular filtration rate may be estimated from the body length and serum creatinine; the respective values are included in Fig. 3.5. Split ^{131}I-hippuran clearance studies were performed in ten children with the Oberhausen (1978) partly-shielded whole body technique. This method permits reliable quantification of unilateral renal plasma flow with a good correlation to invasive para-aminohippuric acid clearance studies with separated urine collections. All parameters were within the normal range (Fig. 3.6).

The Metabolic State

Three patients never needed substitution therapy. In all other children it was administered at 1–13 years; five children are still under treatment. With the exception of the child with ureterosigmoidostomy after cystectomy for rhabdomyosarcoma of the bladder who was not available for this follow-up study, no child had to be readmitted because of a metabolic crisis. The reasons for recurrent

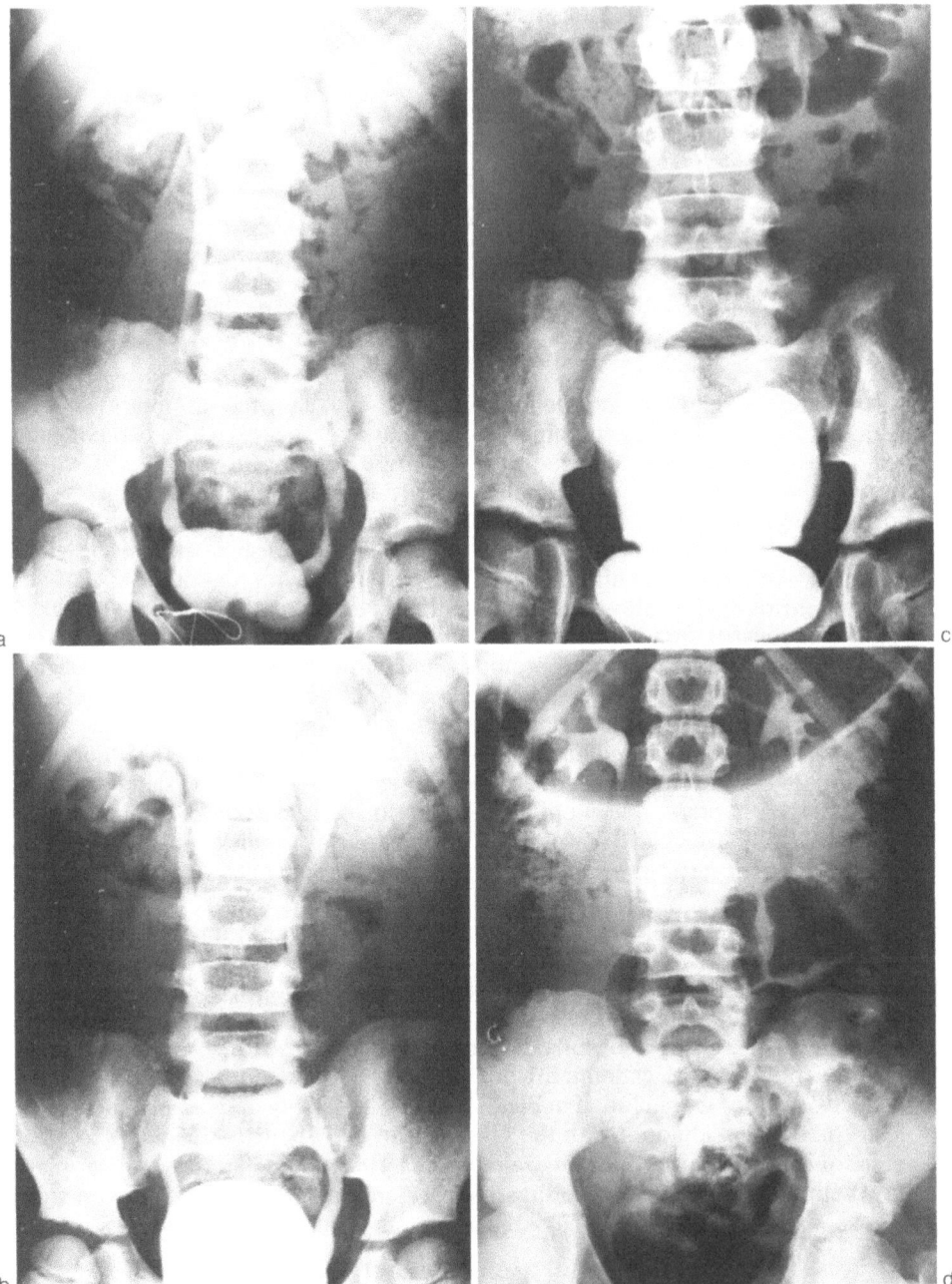

Fig.3.4. A 5-year-old girl, incontinent and obstructed after staged attempt at functional closure of bladder exstrophy. **a** Excretory urogram, pyelonephritic scarring of left kidney. **b** Cystogram, bilateral vesicoureteric reflux. Conversion to ureterosigmoidostomy in spite of scarred left kidney. Asymptomatic and continent since, but metabolic substitution therapy still necessary. **c** Liquid dye enema 2 years after ureterosigmoidostomy; no coloureterial reflux. **d** Excretory urogram 7 years after ureterosigmoidostomy; progressive scarring of left kidney. This is a poor candidate for ureterosigmoidostomy and the author would today rather perform a colonic conduit despite the smooth postoperative course.

hyperchloraemic hypokalaemic acidosis in the tumour child were irregularities of the supplementation treatment following gastro-intestinal complications of chemotherapy; since termination of the adjuvant tumour treatment the child has had no further metabolic problems.

The children occasionally complain of thirst, and all drink plentifully. Figure 3.7 gives the results of the blood gas analyses at the recall examination, and Fig. 3.8 the serum electrolyte values. Metabolic imbalances may therefore be reliably prevented.

Continence

At the time of the last examination, 13 of the 16 children were completely continent day and night, i.e., needed no protective pads at any time. A 12-year-old girl experienced occasional soiling during day or night, in particular in association with liquid stools. Two children were occasionally incontinent at night. Some children, however, did not achieve complete control of urine until their tenth year of life. For years they had appeared to be incontinent and therefore operative failures. The decision to change a ureterosigmoidostomy to a conduit because of incontinence must therefore be delayed until the onset of puberty.

It proved difficult to evaluate the toilet habits of the children, but they did not seem to be upset by this type of urinary diversion. All appeared to participate in the normal social and sporting activities of their contemporaries, and gave the impression of normal childhood. Reliable information on the voiding frequency could not be obtained. In an adult series reinvestigated recently (Marberger et al. to be published), 44% of the patients emptied their rectum an average of once per night, 29% twice, and the rest more frequently. In these patients ureterosigmoidostomy

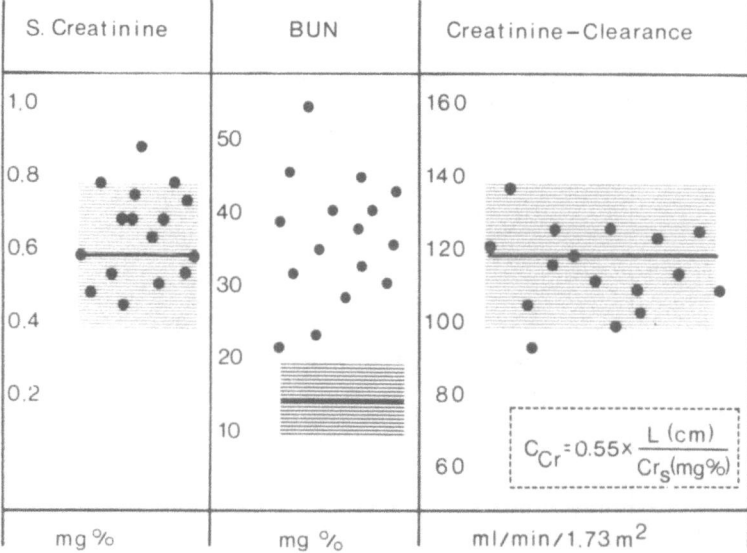

Fig.3.5. Serum BUN, serum creatinine and creatinine clearance calculated according to the Schwartz formula (Schwartz et al. 1976) from the serum creatinine values and body length of the same patients as in Fig. 3.2.

had usually been performed late in life following an ablative procedure for cancer. In the author's opinion, the micturition intervals are significantly longer in children who learn to control their anal sphincter for urine in early childhood. Not one of them, nor their parents, complained of uncomfortable frequency.

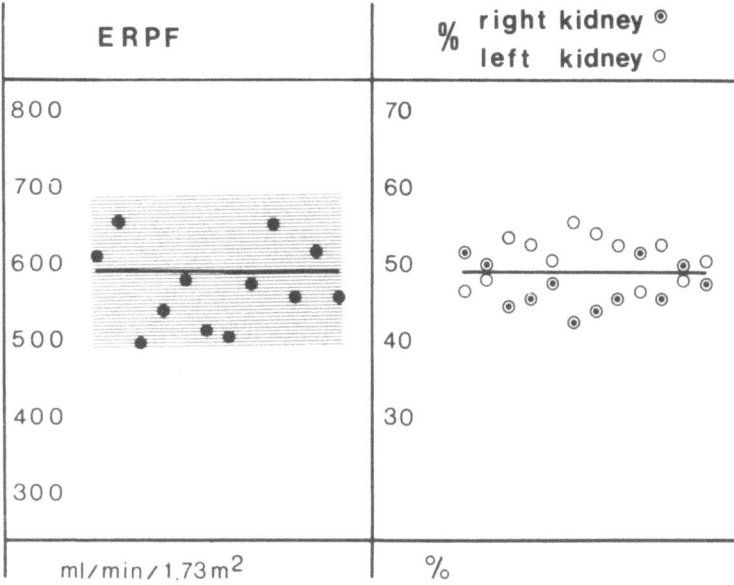

Fig.3.6. Effective renal plasma flow and percentage contributed by the individual kidney as calculated by ^{131}I-hippuran clearance with the Oberhausen technique in 10 patients a mean 10.7 years after ureterosigmoidostomy in childhood (*shaded*, normal range).

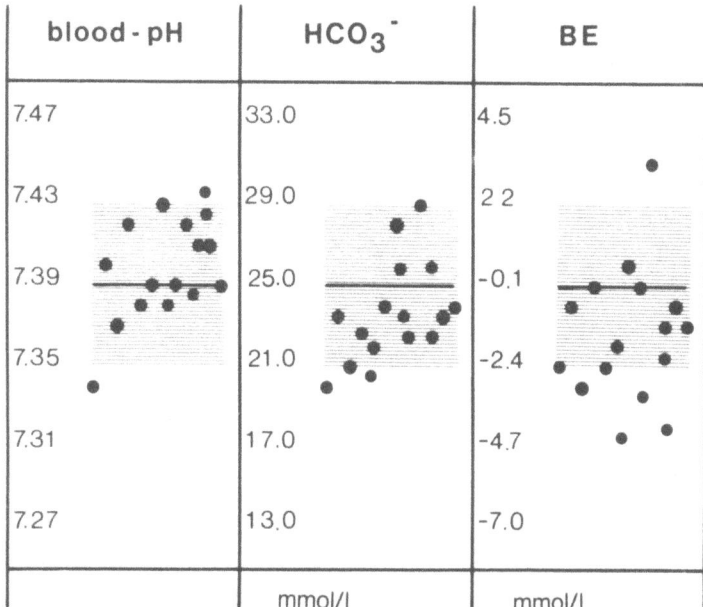

Fig.3.7. Blood gas analysis, same patients as in Fig. 3.2 (*shaded*, normal range).

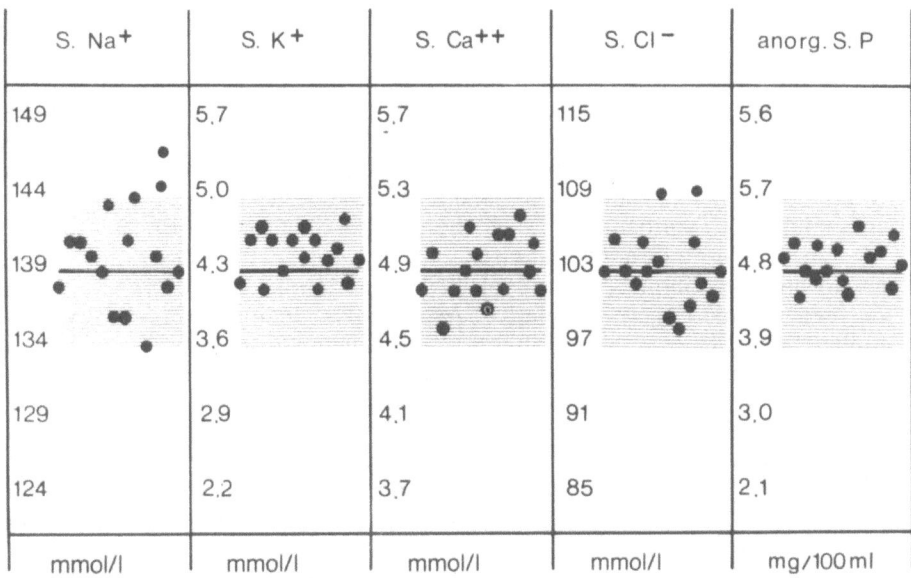

S. Na+	S. K+	S. Ca++	S. Cl⁻	anorg. S. P
149	5.7	5.7	115	5.6
144	5.0	5.3	109	5.7
139	4.3	4.9	103	4.8
134	3.6	4.5	97	3.9
129	2.9	4.1	91	3.0
124	2.2	3.7	85	2.1
mmol/l	mmol/l	mmol/l	mmol/l	mg/100 ml

Fig.3.8. Serum electrolyte values, same patients as in Fig. 3.2 (*shaded*, normal range).

Conversion to Alternative Diversion

In the series reported herein no patient had to be converted. At the University of Mainz Medical School this has, however, become necessary on several occasions among adolescents and adults, as reported elsewhere (Jonas et al. 1980). Renal deterioration with recurrent attacks of acute pyelonephritis and renal lithiasis were the usual indications. An analysis of these patients, however, revealed that the criteria for patient selection for ureterosigmoidostomy had almost always been ignored. Most patients already had a severely damaged upper urinary tract or scarred ureters. In children the largest threat in this direction arises from complications of primary reconstruction of bladder exstrophy. Although incontinence may be the major social problem, obstruction and renal infection are the more dangerous threats of this approach. It must be borne in mind that they may prohibit diversion by ureterosigmoidostomy altogether if reconstruction fails, and may directly require a conduit.

A 16-year-old girl was diverted from a poorly functioning ileal conduit to a ureterosigmoidostomy. Patient and parents considered a stoma unacceptable and denied any previous rectal problems. Although at digital palpation the anal sphincter had appeared weak the patient claimed to hold the saline enema. After uretero-sigmoidostomy she proved to be completely incontinent and had to be converted to a colonic conduit. The parents now disclosed that rectal prolapse had already been corrected at the time of the first diversion. Compromises regarding the prerequisites for ureterosigmoidostomy, in particular concerning anal continence, must be avoided under all circumstances, even under psychological pressure from the patient.

Colonic Tumours and Ureterosigmoidostomy

There is growing evidence of an increased rate of colonic neoplasms in uretero-sigmoidostomy patients. Spence et al. (1978) collected data on 55 patients from the literature with bowel tumours following this type of diversion and added two of their own. Among the 127 patients with ureterosigmoidostomy recently reviewed in Mainz, one 18-year-old had a benign sigmoid polyp 16 years after uretero-sigmoidostomy (Marberger et al. to be published). Characteristically the lesions develop at the ureteric implantation site; three-fourths of the tumours are malignant, usually adenocarcinoma (Pierce et al. 1978). The aetiological factors involved are at the present time largely speculative. As, however, tumours were observed at the implantation site even years after a ureterosigmoidostomy was converted to a conduit, local mechanical trauma around the ureteric orifices by the faecal stream with subsequent metaplasia and transformation of the ureteral mucosa seemed plausible (Spence et al. 1978). The latency period between ureterosigmoidostomy and diagnosis of the tumour varies from 10 to 46 years, with a mean of 25 years (Spence et al. 1978). Pierce et al. (1978) collected data suggesting that the colon of patients older than 40 years might be even more vulnerable to tumour development with a shorter lag period.

Recent interesting research work at both the Peter Bent Brigham Hospital in Boston and the St. Peter's Hospitals in London, has suggested a biochemical explanation for carcinogenesis at the ureterocolic anastomosis. Crissey et al. (1980), using a rat model, have shown that adenocarcinoma close to the ureterocolic anastomosis is prevented by proximal diversion of faeces, implying that faecal carcinogens are activated locally by the urine. Stewart et al. (1981) have postulated a theory of carcinogenesis involving bacterial activation of endogenously formed N-nitrosamine. In a prospective clinical study, preliminary results of rectal urine analysis supports this theory in that high concentrations of N-nitrosamine have been found and mutagens demonstrated (for further discussion see p. 83 Chap. 4).

With a risk of developing a colonic neoplasm 100–500 times greater than in the normal population (Spence et al. 1975; Pierce et al. 1978), this is a grave deficit of ureterosigmoidostomy, and indeed warnings have been issued to completely abandon the procedure in patients with benign disease (Rabinovitch 1980). The present authors consider this premature. Most of the patients reported with colonic neoplasms had their ureterosigmoidostomy performed with the Coffey technique, which leaves a segment of poorly nourished ureter protruding into the colon and therefore subject to considerable local trauma and infiltration. Perhaps the improved anastomotic techniques will reduce the tumour rate. Modern endoscopy techniques permit visualisation of the mucosa with low risk and little inconvenience to the patient, while precise mucosa-mucosa anastomosis definitely shows fewer signs of local irritation (Marberger 1977). Finally, experience with the colonic conduit, alternative of choice to ureterosigmoidostomy, is still too limited to rule out an increased rate of neoplasms in the isolated bowel segment. Nevertheless, all ureterosigmoidostomy patients must be closely monitored for this potential late complication, and with signs of sudden ureteric obstruction or blood in the stool, further diagnostic measures must be undertaken at once.

Conclusion

When considering a ureterosigmoidostomy in a child, it is essential to start with normal upper renal tracts, a healthy colon and continent anal sphincter. The surgical technique should avoid ureteric stenosis and prevent ureteric reflux. There must also be facilities for long term clinical, radiological and metabolic surveillance. This will ensure that there will not be a silent deterioration of the upper renal tracts and renal function, so that ureterosigmoidostomy can be used as an alternative to urinary conduits without the psychological and social burdens of a wet cutaneous stoma.

In bladder exstrophy, the authors consider ureterosigmoidostomy the diversion of choice, provided the upper renal tracts have not deteriorated following earlier attempts at bladder reconstruction and that anal continence is assured. Late malignant change close to the ureterocolic anastomoses remains a worrying danger, but provided the patient's General Practitioner, in addition to the urologist, is aware of this potential complication, it should not outweigh the many advantages of an appliance-free urinary diversion with a stable ureterosigmoidostomy.

References

Alken P, Altwein JE, Jonas U (1978) Transversum conduit — Indikation und Technik. In: Weber W, Jonas D (ed) Reinterventionen an den Urogenitalorganen. Thieme, Stuttgart, pp 59–67

Arap S, Giron AM, DeGoes GM (1980) Initial results of the complete reconstruction of bladder exstrophy. Urol Clin North Am 7: 477–491

Bakker NJ, Cornil C (1974) Techniques and complications of ureterosigmoidostomy and ureterointestinal conduit. In: Johnston JH, Scholtemeijer RJ (eds) Problems in pediatric urology, Excerpta Medica, Amsterdam, pp 91–113

Bettex M (1977) Erfahrungen mit der Harnleiter-Darmtransplantation bei Kindern. In: Zingg E, Tscholl R (eds) Die supravesikale Harnableitung. Huber, Berne Stuttgart Vienna

Boddy K, King PC, Stewart WK, Flemming LW (1975) Whole-body potassium in patients with uretero-sigmoid anastomoses. Br J Urol 47: 277–282

Chisholm GD (1977) Renal function after urinary diversion. In: Zingg E, Tscholl R (eds) Die supra-vesicale Harnableitung. Huber, Berne Stuttgart Vienna, pp 88–94

Clarke BG, Leadbetter WF (1955) Ureterosigmoidostomy: Collective review of results in 2897 reported cases. J Urol 73: 999–1008

Crissey MM, Steele GD, Gittes RF (1980) Rat model for carcinogenesis in ureterosigmoidostomy. Science 207: 1079–1080

Dunn M, Roberts JBM, Smith PJB, Slade N (1979) The long-term results of ileal conduit urinary diversion in children. Br J Urol 51: 458–461

Elder DD, Moisey CV, Rees RWM (1979) A long-term follow-up of the colonic conduit operation in children. Br J Urol 51: 462–465

Goodwin WE, Harris AP, Kaufman JJ, Beal JM (1953) Open transcolonic ureterointestinal anastomosis: A new approach. Surg Gynecol Obstet 97: 282–295

Goodwin WE, Scardino PT (1977) Ureterosigmoidostomy. J Urol 118: 169–174

Heidler H, Marberger M, Hohenfellner R (1979) The metabolic situation in ureterosigmoidostomy. Eur Urol 5: 39–44

Hohenfellner R (1977) Ureterosigmoidostomy. In: Eckstein HB, Hohenfellner R, Williams DI (eds) Surgical pediatric urology. Thieme, Stuttgart, p 354

Hohenfellner R, Marberger M (1980) Film: Ureterosigmoidostomy in children. The AUA-Eaton Film Library

Jonas U, Ferrari B, Hohenfellner R (1980) Sekundäre Harnumleitung nach supravesikaler Harnableitung-Konversion. Acta Urol Belg 11: 317

Koff SA (1975) Mechanism of electrolyte imbalance following urointestinal anastomosis. Urology 5: 109–114

Marberger M (1977) Erfahrungen mit der Harnleiterdarmimplantation. In: Zingg E, Tscholl R (eds) Die supravesikale Harnableitung. Huber, Berne Stuttgart Vienna, p 210

Marberger M, Walz P, Hohenfellner R (to be published) Ureterosigmoidostomy and colonic conduit. Indication, technique and results. J Urol Nephrol (Paris)

Mathiesen W (1953) A new method for ureterointestinal anastomosis. Surg Gynecol Obstet 96: 255–258

Megalli M, Lattimer JK (1973) Review of the management of 140 cases of exstrophy of the bladder. J Urol 109: 246–248

Oberhausen E (1978) Clinical experience with unilateral ^{131}I-hippuran clearances. In: Bianchi CP, Blaufox MD (eds) Unilateral renal function studies. Contributions to nephrology. Karger, Basel, p 22

Pierce EH Jr, Zickerman P, Leadbetter GW Jr (1978) Ureterosigmoidostomy and carcinoma of colon. Trans Am Assoc Genitourin Surg 70: 92

Pinck BD, Alexander S, Siegendorf S (1975) Ureteroileosigmoidostomy. Long-term results. Urology 5: 595–598

Rabinovitch HH (1980) Ureterosigmoidostomy in children — revival or demise? (Guest Editorial) J Urol 124: 552

Schwartz GI, Haycock GB, Edelman CM Jr, Spitzer A (1976) A simple estimate of glomerular filtrate rate in children derived from body length and plasma creatinine. Pediatrics 58: 259–263

Schwarz GR, Jeffs RD (1975) Ileal conduit urinary diversion in children: Computer analysis of follow-up from 2 to 16 years. J Urol 114: 285–288

Shapiro SR, Lebowitz R, Colodny AH (1975) Fate of 90 children with ileal conduit urinary diversion a decade later: Analysis of complications, pyelography, renal function and bacteriology. J Urol 114: 289–295

Spence HM, Hoffman WW, Pate VA (1975) Exstrophy of the bladder. I. Longterm results in a series of 37 cases treated by ureterosigmoidostomy. J Urol 114: 133–137

Spence HM, Hoffman WW, Fosmire GP (1978) Tumour of the colon as a late complication of ureterosigmoidostomy for exstrophy of the bladder. Br J Urol 51: 466–470

Stewart M, Hill MJ, Pugh RCB, Williams JP (1981) The role of N-nitrosamine in carcinogenesis at the ureterocolic anastomosis. Br J Urol 53: 115–118

Walz PH, Alken P (1980) Der Einfluß anatomischer Normvarianten des Sigmas auf die Spätergebnisse der Ureterosigmoidostomie. Acta Urol Belg 11: 161

Zincke H, Segura JW (1975) Ureterosigmoidostomy: Critical review of 173 cases. J Urol 113: 324–327

Chapter 4

Urinary Diversion in Malignant Disease

Anthony Walsh

Two themes run through the whole of this book; be sure that diversion is really indicated and if it is, try to select the diversion most suited to the individual patient. When a bladder must be removed the only problem is to choose the type of diversion but in many patients with advanced malignant disease one must answer the question — is diversion indicated at all? This problem is discussed in detail later in this chapter.

In the past quarter century, the ileal conduit has been the preferred method of diversion in the vast majority of cases but it is now beginning to be realised that there is still no perfect method of urinary diversion. Alternative and older methods are being reconsidered in many major centres. The ileal conduit is discussed in detail in other chapters and it is appropriate to consider the alternatives at this stage.

Colonic Conduit

The colonic conduit was popularised by Mogg (1965) as a method of diversion in children with neuropathic bladder disorders. Mogg claimed that there was far less intraperitoneal manipulation than in the formation of an ileal conduit and that the post-operative course was smoother with less tendency to ileus. He also considered that the colonic conduit would not distend or elongate as ileal conduits do. The chief advantages of the colonic conduit seemed to lie in the reduced risk of stomal stenosis and the much greater possibility of implanting the ureters with an anti-reflux technique. Early reports from other workers were most encouraging and in some centres it came to be preferred to the ileal conduit for diversion in malignant disease. The early promise has not, alas, been fulfilled. Elder et al. (1979) reviewed the results of colonic conduit urinary diversion in 41 children with an average follow-up of 13 years. There was a high incidence of stomal stenosis, uretero-colic stenosis, ureteric reflux and upper tract deterioration. They concluded that comparison with results of ileal conduit diversion in children showed no advantage in the use of colon.

It is probably reasonable at this stage to say that in the context of the patient with malignant disease, a colonic conduit is at least as good as an ileal conduit. In patients who have had radical radiotherapy to the pelvis there is a special place for the use of a transverse colon conduit as described in the section: 'Diversion in the Radiated Patient'.

Long-Term Surveillance

The first essential in all patients with conduits is the availability of a stoma therapist who will not only see that the patient has no problems with appliances but will also check that stomal stenosis is not developing. Indeed, patients who for some reason such as geographic location cannot have access to a stoma therapist should probably not be considered at all for diversion to the abdominal wall, whether by conduit or by cutaneous ureterostomy.

It may not be possible to prevent all complications but serious damage to the upper renal tract can be reduced to a minimum by early corrective surgery. An intravenous urogram and renogram should be done about three months postoperatively. To reduce the total radiation dosage and cost, the intravenous urogram can be limited to one or two films showing the full length of both ureters to check for ureteric obstruction. An annual renogram is the simplest and most sensitive method of follow-up to detect ureteric obstruction. A loopogram need be done only if the intravenous urogram shows ureteric obstruction, or if urinary tract infections become a problem associated with a significant residual urine on catheterising the conduit (Chaps. 2 & 5). If a refluxing uretero-ileal anastomosis has been used, the disappearance of ureteric reflux on the loopogram suggests that there is some ureteric stenosis.

If unilateral ureteric stenosis is demonstrated and confirmed two to three months later, the reimplantation should be repeated. With the Wallace I technique there is a small incidence of ureteric stenosis due to some local mechanical problem at the ureteric anastomosis and occasionally the terminal left ureter develops an ischaemic stricture following mobilisation of the ureter behind the pelvic mesocolon to the right iliac fossa. No long-term results are available for the incidence of ureteric stenosis using the Wallace II technique.

On re-exploration, the procedure will depend on the operative findings. In some cases, the obstructed ureter is reimplanted separately into the conduit, whilst in others the obstructed ureter is anastomosed end to side into the free draining ureter.

To avoid risking stenosis at the ureteroileal anastomosis, Clark (1979) recommends a Y anastomosis with spatulation of the ureters which are then joined to form a single tube and anastomosed to the end of the ileum. Clark's results are 'almost as good as the best obtained with the Bricker operation, and better than many reported series' (Fig. 4.1).

It is often thought that biochemical disorders are insignificant in patients with conduits. This is not necessarily so (Castro and Ram 1970) and a full biochemical screen should be carried out at each yearly review.

Ureterosigmoidostomy

As the preferred method of urinary diversion, ureterosigmoidostomy reached its apogee shortly after 1950. Then came Bricker and the ileal conduit. The conduit was accepted with enthusiasm as a much better method of diversion and by 1970 there were very few urologists who did not regard it as the only method for urinary diversion. In the past decade there has been a growing awareness of the considerable complications, early and late, associated with conduits; Schmidt et al. (1973) reviewed 178 consecutive patients subjected to ileal diversion from 1961 to 1969. In the 48 cases who had diversion carried out for malignant disease, there was a 50%

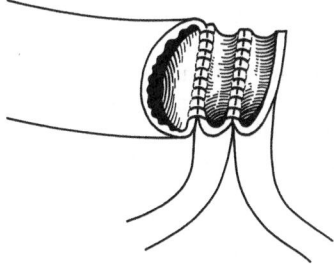

Wallace I 1966

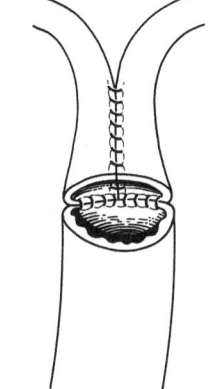

Y anastomosis, Clark 1979

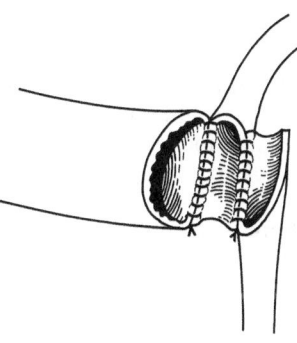

Wallace II 1970

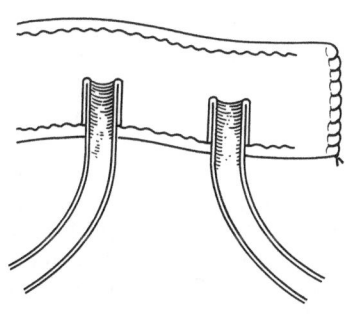

Nipple anastomosis

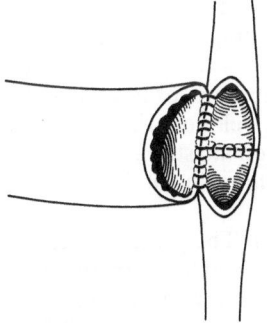

Modified Wallace

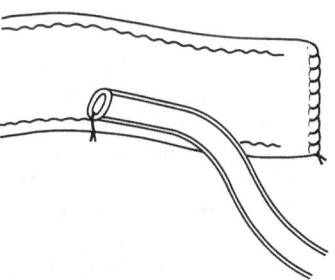

'Drop in' anastomosis

Fig.4.1. A choice of current techniques for ureteroileal anastomoses.

incidence of both early and late complications. In the entire series, complications treated by non-surgical means necessitated 114 patient admissions. Secondary surgical procedures for complications were indicated in 147 instances. Only 32 patients (19%) in the series had no complications. Other authors reported similar experience and this led to a reappraisal of ureterosigmoidostomy.

A critical review of all the complications encountered in 173 patients who underwent ureterosigmoidostomy at the Mayo Clinic between 1957 and 1966 was undertaken by Zincke and Segura (1975). Eighty per cent of the operations were performed for malignant disease. It is worth quoting their conclusion: 'The procedure has much to recommend from a patient's standpoint, including absence of a stoma, none of the problems of an external collecting device and the quasi-normal form of urinary control. From the surgeon's standpoint the somewhat simpler operating technique and definitely shorter operating time seemed to be distinct advantages. Furthermore, conversion to another form of diversion may be accomplished at a later date if necessary. We do not mean to imply that use of ileal conduit diversion should be abandoned. However, we think that ureterosig-moidostomy compares favourably with ileal conduit diversion and that it should be considered more frequently as the method of diversion.'

In order to make a rational appreciation of the proper role of ureterosig-moidostomy at the present time, we must consider in detail the possible hazards, problems and complications. There are two main sources of trouble: (1) Technical errors in the anastomosis of the ureters to the colon; and (2) Biochemical disorders initiated by the absorption of urine constituents from the colon.

1) Technical errors in uretero-colic anastomosis: If there is any interference with the blood supply of the ureter, the anastomosis to the colon may break down with a consequent leak of urine and faecal matter, a complication that may easily prove fatal in a debilitated patient struggling to recover from major surgery. The key to avoiding this complication is to mobilise the ureter as little as possible. The bowel should be brought to the ureter and not the ureter to the bowel. Some mobilisation of the ureter is unavoidable and here we must apply the lessons learnt in kidney transplantation. The higher the ureter can be divided the better. Mobilisation should be carried out by dissecting at least 1 cm away from the wall of the ureter to minimise the risk of damage to the longitudinal anastomotic vessels. The posterior parietal peritoneum should be incised carefully over the ureter so that the ureter will run in a smooth curve to the colon without any angulation. The sigmoid colon should be fixed to the posterior peritoneum so that there will be no drag or tension on the anastomosis.

Any narrowing, stricture or stenosis of the ureter will cause upper tract dilatation and this will inevitably be complicated by ascending pyelonephritis and often secondary stone formation. On the other hand, a wide open anastomosis will allow free reflux of faecal material up the ureter with the same inevitable result of pyelonephritis and progressive destruction of the kidney.

A great many techniques have been proposed (Fig. 4.2). The principal methods were very well summarised by Jacobs (1953). In the Coffey and Stiles methods, the ureter was led in to the colon and its tip then anchored to the bowel wall, leaving 2–3 cm of terminal ureter free in the lumen of the gut. These methods were very liable to obstruction from angulation or fibrosis of the ureter at its site of entry into the bowel lumen, stenosis of the ureter by scar tissue in the course of its passage through the bowel wall and stricture at the tip of the ureteral stump lying within the bowel lumen. The direct methods of Nesbit (1949) and Cordonnier (1949) were devised to minimise or eliminate these risks by performing a careful mucosa-to-mucosa anastomosis. The

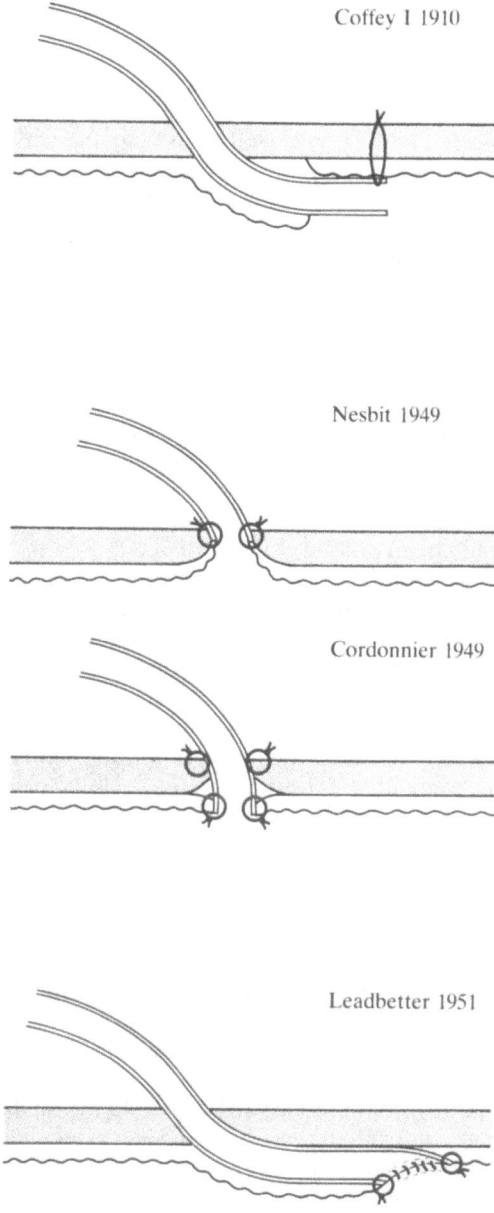

Fig.4.2. Techniques for ureterosigmoidostomy.

Cordonnier technique was a direct end-to-side anastomosis of a dilated ureter to the colon, with a single layer of interrupted chromic catgut sutures. The Nesbit technique was similar but applicable to ureters of normal calibre; the end of the ureter was spatulated and then anastomosed to a small opening in the colon using interrupted catgut sutures through the full thickness of the walls of the ureter and colon. Nesbit and Cordonnier were right in their emphasis on the importance of accurate mucosal approximation but the absence of any valve mechanism allowed free reflux of bowel content up the ureters — in the long run just as disastrous as the stricture problems inherent in the older techniques. The advantages of the submucous tunnel advocated by Coffey and the direct anastomoses proposed by Nesbit and Cordonnier were combined by Leadbetter (1951). He made an incision, 2.5 cm long, slightly diagonally across the anterior taenia of the colon from the mesenteric margin of the bowel. A trough was created in the bowel wall by incising the various layers down to the mucosa itself and gently stripping the mucosa away from the overlying muscularis, thus forming generous flaps on either side. Leadbetter laid great emphasis on the importance of carrying the incision in the bowel right down to the mucosal layer. He believed that, if this were not done properly, the ureter lay between relatively non-yielding sub-mucosa and resutured muscle layers whereas, when properly performed, the mucosa acted as a hammock which invaginated into the bowel and so avoided constriction of the ureter. This is accomplished by incising the layers of the bowel wall very carefully at the distal end of the trough until the mucosa is identified, sometimes by actually perforating it. The incision can then be dissected back within the proper layer. The dissection is carried all the way to the mesenteric margin of the bowel so that the ureter is subsequently led directly into the trough. On the left side it is usually convenient to pass the ureter through an opening in the sigmoid mesocolon. A short opening is made through the mucosa at the distal end of the trough (if one has not already been produced in the dissection) and then the spatulated end of the ureter is anastomosed carefully to the bowel mucosa. Leadbetter used fine silk sutures but it is wiser to use 4/0 or 5/0 chromic catgut. The muscular flaps of the bowel wall are then stitched loosely over the ureter and here we prefer to follow Leadbetter's practice of using interrupted silk sutures. It is absolutely essential that the entry of the ureter into the tunnel is not tight and when the anastomosis has been completed the looseness of the tunnel should be tested by passing a small haemostat into it. Anyone not familiar with the technique would do well to read Leadbetter's excellent original description of the details of the procedure.

It is now generally agreed that the combination of an anti-reflux tunnel with direct anastomosis is the only acceptable method of uretero-colic diversion. The same object was achieved by Goodwin et al. (1953). They considered that it was easier to perform an accurate anastomosis by opening the colon along its anti-mesenteric border and creating a tunnel close to the mesenteric border by blunt dissection — then at the upper end of the tunnel making an opening close to the mesentery by passing through a curved haemostat which was used to draw the ureter in along the tunnel to the bowel. The mucosa-to-mucosa anastomosis could then be performed very easily under direct vision.

One of the advantages of this technique is that it is easy to place a stent, usually a 6F tube of PVC or Silastic. There is a great deal to be said for using stents whenever urine is diverted to the bowel as a single stage procedure at the same time as a radical cystectomy (as is the normal practice). There is always some oedema at the site of the anastomosis for a few days, producing some degree of ureteric obstruction and therefore impairment of kidney function, at the very time that the kidneys have to deal with the big metabolic load of major pelvic surgery. The stents should provide free drainage of urine in the critical first few days after operation. If the ureteric stents are brought out through the anal canal and anchored to the perianal skin, differential urine outputs from the two kidneys can be measured. If these catheters drain well it obviates the need for a rectal catheter and so avoids stretching the anal sphincter which may at least temporarily compromise full rectal continence. These stents are removed by gentle traction about the tenth post-operative day if healing appears uneventful. It is a great mistake to put in a relatively short stent draining into the rectum with no method of direct retrieval in the hope that it will soon be passed down to the lower rectum; instead of being passed downwards, the stent can migrate upwards! On such an occasion after waiting in vain for its elimination, we had to remove it from the ureter by open surgery six weeks later.

An ingenious modification of the Goodwin technique was devised by Hohenfellner (1977). Here again the site of the anastomosis is exposed through an anterior incision in the sigmoid colon. After removing a small button-hole in the posterior wall of the colon, the ureters are brought in to the lumen along a tunnel just beneath the peritoneum of the meso-sigmoid. A submucosal tunnel of about 3 cm in length is then made in the posterior sigmoid wall between stay sutures and the ureter threaded through. The ureter is spatulated and approximated accurately to the intestinal mucosa with interrupted 5/0 chromic catgut sutures, with the most distal suture going through the muscle wall of the colon as an anchor stitch. Good results with this technique have been reported by Marberger et al. (Chap. 3, p. 60).

There is always the possibility that this form of diversion may later need to be revised to separate the urine and the faeces and it makes sense to plan the ureterosigmoidostomy so that its conversion will be relatively simple — either as a rectosigmoid bladder with a colostomy or to a colonic conduit. This is what Turner-Warwick (1976) has called a three-option diversion (Fig. 4.3). The ureters are implanted into the colon in such a way that subsequent conversion does not need much revision of the pedicle or reimplantation of the ureters.

2) Biochemical disorders: The disturbances of body chemistry following ureterosigmoidostomy have been known for 25 years or more (Stamey 1956). The problems

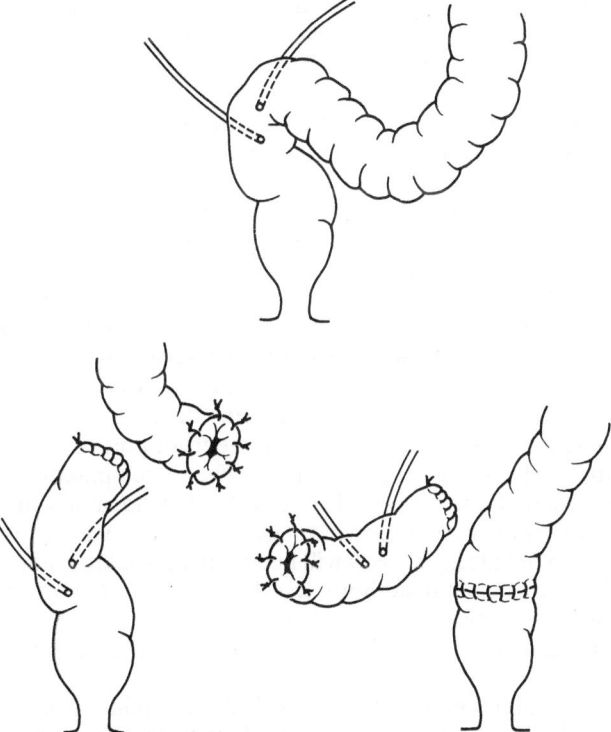

Fig.4.3. 'Three-option' ureterosigmoid diversion (Turner-Warwick).

are caused by absorption of chloride and ammonium ions and urea from the urine and by a loss of potassium. Late pyelogram films after ureterosigmoidostomy show that, no matter how low the implantation of the ureters, urine may wash back all the way to the caecum so that absorption takes place from the entire colonic mucosa. Put simply, the absorbed chloride displaces bicarbonate, producing the well known hyperchloraemic acidosis. The absorbed water and urea probably do little more than promote diuresis but the absorbed urea causes a rise in plasma urea level which may be misinterpreted as evidence of depressed renal function. This error of inter-pretation can be avoided by measuring serum creatinine because creatinine is not absorbed from the bowel. Ammonium may be formed from the urinary urea by urea-splitting bacteria in the bowel. The ammonium is absorbed with chloride and so, as pointed out by Chisholm (1977), the steady infusion of urine into the bowel is equivalent to a steady infusion of ammonium chloride into the circulation. In patients with normal renal function, the kidneys are able to compensate and serious acidosis seldom develops but, if renal function is depressed, the acidosis may prove a serious threat to life. It is for this reason that ureterosigmoidostomy should be considered as a method of diversion only in patients with normal kidney function. Even where kidney function is normal at the time of surgery, problems can arise as a result of ascending pyelonephritis or if the patient should become dehydrated in any acute intercurrent illness. The family doctor who looks after the patient must be alerted to these dangers.

It is sometimes suggested that, when the urine has been diverted into the intact colon, salt intake should be restricted. It is certainly reasonable to counsel the patient against excessive salt intake but the restriction should not be too severe. Excessive salt restriction may affect renal function and, furthermore, it renders food very unpalatable and this in turn may lead to anorexia. If a patient with uretero-sigmoidostomy does present acutely ill with severe hyperchloraemic acidosis, continuous rectal tube drainage will almost eliminate the abnormalities due to absorption.

Potassium loss may be very important. Irritation of the colon by urine may produce an excessive amount of secretion with a high potassium content. This is similar to the potassium loss in patients with papillomata of the colon and in chronic laxative abuse. The problem may be compounded by hyperchloraemic acidosis which leads to increased renal excretion of potassium. Furthermore, chronic pyelonephritis can cause excessive potassium loss from the kidneys and in turn the hypokalaemia causes renal tubular dysfunction so that a vicious circle is set up. At post-mortem examination of patients dying after ureterocolic anastomosis, Stamey (1956) found that 17 of 57 patients had vacuolation in the proximal tubules.

As shown by Williams et al. (1967), a depletion in whole body potassium is to be expected in patients with ureterocolic anastomosis and this depletion may not be reflected in the plasma potassium concentrations. Supplements of potassium citrate may be advisable from the early post-operative period. The development of any acute gastro-intestinal disease with loss of bowel content by diarrhoea or vomiting and the resultant potassium loss may precipitate hypokalaemic states out of proportion to the loss. Such hypokalaemic crises will need infusion of large amounts of potassium to replace the body deficit in addition to other measures to correct the electrolyte imbalance. It is our practice to give oral potassium citrate to all patients with ureterosigmoidostomy and we try to keep the plasma potassium above 4 mmol/l.

It will be obvious from the foregoing that blood levels of creatinine, potassium, electrolytes and acid–base balance must be monitored daily in the early post-operative period. In addition, it is wise to minimise colonic absorption at this early stage. If the ureteric stents do not drain urine well a 24F Foley catheter is inserted into the rectum for 3–4 days.

Osteomalacia

This is an occasional late complication of ureterosigmoidostomy. There is a good deal of evidence in the literature that the osteomalacia is secondary to metabolic acidosis. Lee et al. (1977) have shown that the conversion of 25 hydroxychole-calciferol to 1,25 dihydroxycholecalciferol is inhibited by metabolic acidosis. The earliest symptoms of osteomalacia are bone pain, weakness and muscle stiffness. Such symptoms occurring in the patient whose urine has been diverted to the colon are an indication for full biochemical and radiological study. The diagnosis may be confirmed by iliac crest biopsy. The osteomalacia will heal in a matter of months when the acidosis is corrected by the oral administration of sodium bicarbonate and potassium citrate. There is no point in giving Vitamin D as well because the condition is Vitamin D resistant. In view of the work of Winterborn et al. (1978) it would seem unwise to give 1α-hydroxycholecalciferol because it may lead to hypercalcaemia and to deterioration of renal function.

Problems of Urinary Control

Most people who require diversion of urine for malignant disease are in the older age groups. Quite a significant number of such people do not have adequate tone in the levator ani muscles and anal sphincters to ensure full control of fluid in the rectum. Such people should not have the urine diverted to the bowel. The ability to hold fluid should be tested by running 200 ml of water into the rectum through a small tube. The patient should be able to hold this water for at least one and preferably two hours while up and about. Even though they may pass this test, some patients will be found to leak urine at night. This problem can often be solved by giving 25 or 50 mg of imipramine shortly before the patient goes to bed. In a very few cases we have found it necessary to use an enuresis buzzer alarm system or to have the patient use an alarm clock to wake up during the night to void urine.

Hohenfellner recommends checking for nocturnal incontinence by running 200 ml of fluid into the rectum shortly before the patient goes to sleep. This fluid should be retained four to five hours without soiling.

Carcinoma of the Colon as a Late Complication (See also Chap. 3)

It is now well recognised that the risk of developing carcinoma of the colon is at least 100 times greater in patients with uretero-colic anastomosis than in the population at large. The average interval between ureterosigmoidostomy and the diagnosis of the bowel neoplasm is 25 years. The shortest interval reported is ten years, in the first case described in the literature (Hammer 1929). Hammer's case is not entirely typical. His patient had undergone a Maydl type operation for exstrophy at the age of 40 and ten years later died with bowel and uraemic symptoms. Autopsy disclosed a colloid tumour originating from the trigone which had been transposed to the bowel.

The very long interval before the carcinoma develops might suggest that this complication is of little significance in patients who had the urine diverted for malignant disease. However, Spence et al. (1979) collected a total of 55 cases from the literature and in nine of these the original diversion had been performed for bladder cancer. Stewart et al. (1981) traced the notes of 78 patients who underwent ureterocolic diversion for benign disease at St. Peter's Hospital, London, and found seven cases of colonic tumour occurring between 15 and 40 years after diversion.

The tumour is nearly always an adenocarcinoma occurring at the site of anastomosis. Some patients have developed adenomatous polyps. Stewart et al. make the interesting point that the interval after diversion was six years shorter when polyps were diagnosed and they suggest that if adenomatous colonic polyps were to undergo malignant change, it would not be unreasonable that this process would take place over a period of 5–10 years. Stewart et al. produced an interesting hypothesis to explain the development of these colonic tumours. The total dietary nitrate is excreted by the kidneys into the urine. When the urine is diverted to the colon where there is a mixed bacterial flora, we might expect the formation and activation of large amounts of nitroso compounds. N-nitrosamine is a powerful carcinogen to which no laboratory animal has yet proved resistant. These authors have analysed rectal urine collected from patients with ureterosigmoidostomies and have found uniformly raised levels of nitrite, nitrate and N-nitrosamine and have also demonstrated mutagens. This finding is highly significant in that N-nitrosamines are not normally found, in other than trace amounts, in either human faeces or urine. In fact, N-nitrosamines have been demonstrated in only two other locations in the human body — firstly, in the achlorhydric stomach where they have been associated with gastric cancer, and secondly, in the mixed urinary infection associated with bilharzia where, again, they have been incriminated in local carcinogenesis. They conclude that it would be difficult to deny the significance of the demonstration of these compounds in rectal urines, particularly in association with the presence of mutagens.

The hypothesis is very attractive but it is curious that in one of the cases reported by Spence et al. (1979), a boy underwent bilateral ureterosigmoidostomy at the age of three months. Nine months later the diversion was changed to an ileal conduit but 14 years later he developed a colonic carcinoma at the site of the anastomosis. Spence et al. note that at least five patients have developed cancer at the anastomotic site many years after diversion of the urine away from the colon.

Whatever the explanation, the clinical observations and implications are clear and definite. There is a very significant risk of late development of carcinoma of the colon. In the cases reported in the literature, the mortality from cancer in patients with this complication has been very high. It is mandatory, therefore, that the conscientious follow-up of patients who have undergone ureterosigmoid diversion should include a colonoscopy (as far as the uretero-colic anastomoses) every year from about the tenth year onwards. This examination need not be extended more than a short distance above the site of the uretero-colic anastomosis but the endoscopist should be aware of the type of anastomosis: we know of one case in which nipple anastomoses were mistaken for polypoid growths and excised!

Spence et al. (1979) emphasise that whenever one of these patients requires nephrectomy or revision of the uretero-colic anastomosis, it is very important to remove the ureteric stump completely and also the colonic tissue around the orifice.

Patient Selection

It is clear that patients should not be considered for ureterosigmoidostomy unless they have normal kidneys with normal function and also normal ureters. They must also be able to hold fluid in the rectum. Diverticulitis and radiation-induced proctitis are also contra-indications to this method of diversion. Provided that selection along these lines is rigid, ureterosigmoidostomy should probably be the first choice in many patients who need urinary diversion for malignant disease. It is perhaps worth drawing attention to the work of Daniel (Daniel and Ram 1965), who found that intracolonic pressure varied a great deal from one individual to another. Where this pressure exceeded 30 cm of water there was a much higher risk of ascending pyelonephritis and serious complications following ureterocolic anastomosis. He suggested that the special problems associated with high pressure colons might be overcome by performing sigmoid myotomy (Reilly's operation). In our view, this is not to be recommended because it is virtually impossible to perform Reilly's operation without producing several holes in the mucosa, clearly undesirable in the context of uretero-colic anastomosis. This opinion does not, however, detract from the significance of Daniel's observations. His findings were reported at a time when ureterosigmoidostomy had been almost entirely superseded by the use of conduits and this may explain why his work does not seem to have been followed up. If, as many believe, the time has come to restore ureterosigmoidostomy to the repertoire of the urologist, it might be very valuable if Daniel's findings could be confirmed because this might add yet another criterion to patient selection.

Long-Term Surveillance

With this, as with all forms of diversion, the progress of the patients must be monitored for as long as they live. There never comes a time when one can safely say that all is well and further observation is not necessary. Two of our patients were found to have an obstructed uretero-colic anastomosis 19 and 23 years respectively after surgery.

Biochemical screening should include creatinine, urea, full electrolyte and acid–base studies in the blood. If the patient remains well, these tests should be performed 1 month after discharge from hospital, then 3-monthly for 1 year, thereafter twice a year for 5 years. Many workers feel that after 5 years, biochemical screening is necessary only once a year but it is probably safer to continue to do these tests at 6-month intervals.

X-ray studies should ordinarily be limited to two films, a control plain film and a single film, full length, intravenous urogram taken about 30 minutes after injection of contrast medium. We routinely do these X-ray studies at 1, 6 and 12 months and then once every year. If at any stage a kidney fails to excrete the contrast medium, antegrade pyelography is indicated.

If the patient survives for 10 years, colonoscopy should be performed yearly thereafter.

Bone pain, weakness or muscle stiffness are indications, as described above, for a full study to determine the presence or absence of osteomalacia.

Any acute illness, however long after diversion, is an indication for full study. It is absolutely essential that the patient's general practitioner is fully informed on these matters. We have more than once had the unhappy experience of learning that one of our patients had died from a treatable complication of uretero-colic anastomosis in circumstances where for one reason or another the patient's own doctor was not fully aware of all the implications of the diversion. Many of the problems of adequate supervision can be lessened if the patient also is fully informed.

Isolated Recto-Sigmoid Bladder

The rectum and sigmoid colon, isolated from the faecal pathway by terminal iliac colostomy, may be a good bladder substitute. Technically, the operation is relatively simple. It lends itself to staging in the poor risk patient. Because the area of mucosa available for absorption is very much less, there is not the same tendency to hyperchloraemic acidosis as with diversion to the intact colon. For this reason, the isolated recto-sigmoid can be used in patients with moderately defective renal function or with dilated ureters. The risk of ascending pyelonephritis is much less than with diversion to the intact colon. Compared with a conduit or direct cutaneous ureterostomy, the obvious difference is that between a urostomy and a colostomy. The psycho-social implications of the alternative stomata are fundamental in making a choice between the recto-sigmoid bladder and the much more widely used conduit. Faeces naturally excite a far greater repugnance than urine and so there is an obvious tendency to regard a urostomy as more acceptable than a colostomy. This is probably a valid assumption for people living in developed communities with access to good stoma therapy. The situation may be very different for the millions who live in poorer circumstances. A urostomy requires a fairly sophisticated appliance with good facilities for appliance replacement and adjustment. In the absence of such facilities, a colostomy may be far preferable to a leaking, poorly managed urostomy. Ghoneim and Ashamallah (1974) have found the isolated recto-sigmoid bladder to be particularly suitable as the first choice method of diversion when performing cystectomy for bladder carcinoma in Egypt. These authors reported that over 90% of their surviving patients were active, working and socially acceptable. Pyrah (1963) stated: 'The most striking feature of all is the very high grade of health that patients enjoyed provided the malignant disease had not recurred.'

Obviously, as with the intact colon, this mode of diversion can be considered only in patients who are shown to be able to hold water in the rectum. When this condition has been fulfilled, it is rare to find a problem with loss of urine control in the daytime, but up to 40% of patients may experience some incontinence during sleep.

Shehab El Din (1979), working in Ghoneim's department at Mansoura University in Egypt, carried out a controlled trial of imipramine in 40 patients with recto-sigmoid bladders who had nocturnal enuresis. He found an excellent response to imipramine in a dose of 25 mg three times a day. We also have found imipramine very valuable in treating this complication. In our experience it suffices to give 25 or 50 mg of imipramine before the patient goes to bed. We have found a satisfactory response to imipramine in about 70% of patients in whom it was tried (see p. 83). Ghoneim et al. (1981) also favour a submucosal tunnel ureterorectal anastomosis to prevent ureteric reflux.

Hyperchloraemic Acidosis

This occurs in patients with an isolated recto-sigmoid bladder, especially if renal function is impaired, but in our experience this has never proved to be a serious problem. Only a few of our patients have needed to take oral alkali. Two required potassium supplements, given in the form of oral potassium citrate.

Ascending Pyelonephritis

This may complicate some 12% of cases (Ghoneim and Ashamallah 1974). The commonest predisposing factor is stricture or other obstruction at the uretero-sigmoid junction. The rectal urine becomes sterile in about 30% of patents but remains infected in 70%. This raises the question of the significance of reflux. It is commonly held that reflux is not important with this method of diversion but there is now good evidence to the contrary. Shehab El Din (1979) studied 61 patients with invasive bladder carcinoma who were submitted to radical cystectomy and rectal bladder diversion with terminal colostomy as a single stage procedure. In this series one ureter was implanted by a direct technique with no tunnel and the other ureter was placed in a tunnel by the technique described by Goodwin et al. (1953). The subsequent fate of the kidneys was studied by intravenous urography. Significantly more kidneys deteriorated when the anastomosis was direct. There was objective evidence of improvement in renal status following a sub-mucous tunnel technique in 77%, while with the direct technique there was improvement in only 53%. It is certainly very important to avoid stenosis but in our view a tunnel should be used — with either a Leadbetter or a Goodwin technique.

Patient Selection

Patients in whom the only contra-indication to ureterosigmoidostomy is impairment of renal function or ureteric dilatation are the most obvious candidates for this form of diversion. In such cases, the decision lies between colostomy and urostomy, and here one must take into account the personal and social circumstances, including adequate access to stoma therapy, and the patient's own preference. The stoma therapist should have a say in the decision. The patient must be able to hold fluid in the rectum. Diverticulitis in the lower sigmoid colon and radiation proctitis are obvious contra-indications.

The isolated recto-sigmoid bladder is particularly suitable in the very old, poor risk patient if it seems desirable to perform diversion and cystectomy in separate stages.

Follow-up should be exactly the same as in patients with ureterosigmoidostomy.

Combination with Continent Perineal Colostomy

The concept of combining an isolated rectal bladder with a sigmoid colostomy brought down inside the anal sphincters is an attractive one. It offers the prospect of an artificial bladder with voluntary control of urine and faeces. Gersuny (1898) brought the sigmoid colon out anterior to the anal canal whereas in the procedure described by Heitz-Boyer and Hovelacque (1912) the sigmoid colon is brought to the surface in the perineum beneath the internal and external anal sphincters by creating a tunnel behind the rectum in the hollow of the sacrum. From time to time there have been reports of one or other of these procedures used in some half dozen cases. For example, Ensor et al. (1970) reported on a modified Gersuny procedure while Culp and Flocks (1966) and Vereecken et al. (1980) reported their experience of the Heitz-Boyer Hovelacque operation. It has always seemed significant to the present writer that none of the centres that reported some good results went on to report a large series of satisfactory cases. The snag with both methods seems to be the absence of the anal sensation which has a considerable role in normal faecal continence. The procedure should not be attempted in the old, the feeble or in patients with a very limited expectation of life. Like the continent bowel reservoirs described in Chap. 6 these procedures should be attempted only in relatively young patients with a good prognosis.

Culp and Flocks (1966) prefer the Heitz-Boyer Hovelacque procedure because they suggest that, in contrast to the Gersuny technique, it may be hoped that the proprioceptive impulses initiated by stretching the internal rectal sphincter will aid in securing more adequate faecal control. Vereecken et al. (1980) discuss the value of special investigations such as electromanometry. Perhaps the most practical reason for preferring the Heitz-Boyer Hovelacque to the Gersuny procedure is that the latter will often not be feasible in women whose perineal body has been damaged by childbirth.

Cutaneous Ureterostomy

Cutaneous ureterostomy is perhaps the simplest and safest of all methods of permanent urinary diversion. This form of diversion has been used for a very long time but never became popular because of a number of problems and complications, including:

1) Difficulty in fitting a collecting appliance,
2) Stomal stenosis necessitating intubation,
3) Sepsis and stone formation secondary to intubation, and
4) Necrosis of the ureter due to loss of its blood supply during mobilization.

In recent times, most of these objections have been met by improved technique and better selection of cases. It is worth quoting at some length the opinion of Milroy et al. (1978) who reviewed 84 patients managed with cutaneous ureterostomy during the previous 18 years. They concluded: 'many attributes commend the use of the procedure, including the absence of abdominal complications relating to bowel or ureteroenteric anastomoses, the absence of augmentation of electrolyte difficulties engendered by previously existing impaired renal function and intestinal segment electrolyte absorption, the surgical ease of treating stomal stenosis and the availability of ureters for catheterization should the need arise. Furthermore, the incidence of late urographic deterioration (10%) and stone formation (3%) is lower than that often reported for the ileal conduit'. It is worth considering in detail the problems listed above.

1) Difficulty in fitting a collecting appliance has been overcome by improved appliances and above all by appreciation of the importance of choosing the correct site for the stoma. The latter consideration is paramount. It is essential that the site for the stoma be chosen by an experienced stoma therapist. Whether one or both ureters are diverted this way there should be a single stoma.

2) Stomal stenosis in our experience has ceased to be a major problem since we adopted the principles advocated by Lapides (1962) (see Fig. 2.9). For the single

ureter, a U-shaped skin flap is cut at the site of the stoma. The end of the ureter is slit for 2–2.5 cm. The skin flap is sutured in to this slit, using 4/0 chromic catgut with the knots away from the lumen. If there are two ureters with a dilated ureter on one side and a normal sized ureter on the opposite side, the dilated ureter is brought out as just described and the normal ureter is anastomosed to it as a transuretero-ureterostomy. An alternative possibility if both ureters are very dilated is a bilateral cutaneous ureterostomy through a single stoma in which case a Z-plasty is outlined on the skin in the previously selected stomal site and the two ureters are brought out side by side.

We prefer the version of the Lapides technique described by Straffon et al. (1970). Any excess ureter is cut off about 2 cm above the skin level and a longitudinal incision is made in the lateral border of each ureter. The skin flaps of the Z-plasty are then sutured in to the incision made in the ureter using interrupted 4/0 chromic sutures. The mid-point of each ureter opposite the longitudinal incision is sutured to the base of the opposite skin flap and the ureters are approximated to the skin margin with interrupted 4/0 chromic sutures. This leaves one side of each ureter contiguous to the other and they are simply sutured together with a running stitch of 4/0 chromic catgut.

Using these Lapides techniques, we have encountered stomal stenosis only twice in the last 30 cases. In both cases the stenosis was easily dealt with by teaching the patient to use a simple dilator. At least one of these two stenoses was due to faulty technique: it was obvious that the U-flap of skin was lying flat on the abdominal wall and was not properly turned down a sufficient distance in to the ureter. In this last patient the stomal stenosis came to light because the patient formed a series of stones in the ureter. These stones were easily removed with a Dormia basket.

Obstruction higher up the ureter can be a greater nuisance than stomal problems. The ureter may be angled sharply around a fascial edge. It is important to take care to avoid this and to ensure that the ureter runs in a smooth curve on its way to the anterior abdominal wall. In transureteroureterostomy, the same applies to the ureter being brought across from the opposite side.

Another source of obstruction of the ureter is extrinsic stricture where it passes through the abdominal wall or obstruction by a shuttering effect. Again, these problems stem from faulty technique in making the ureterostomy. After the flap or flaps have been raised for the stoma, a cylinder of tissue must be removed from the full thickness of the abdominal wall. The size of this opening through the anterior abdominal wall will obviously depend on the size of the ureter or ureters but in general for one ureter it should accommodate one finger easily and when the ureters are very dilated it should accommodate two fingers.

3) Infection and stone formation secondary to intubation were very common problems when the only material available was rubber. With modern materials these complications should be very much less, as is shown by the success of the Gibbons stent.

4) Sloughing of the ureter through loss of its blood supply during mobilisation is by far the most serious complication of cutaneous ureterostomy. This disaster is generally held to be very common if the ureter is of normal calibre. If a normal ureter is divided very close to the bladder and the pelvic and abdominal ureter are then extensively mobilised, the last few centimeters of ureter are extremely likely to lose their blood supply. However, if the ureter is divided where it crosses the iliac vessels and mobilised with great care to keep at least 1 cm away from the ureter so that the long anastomotic vessels are not compromised, normal ureters can often be used quite successfully as shown by the experience of preserving the blood supply to the ureters in kidney transplantation.

Even greater safety can be achieved with normal ureters by dividing the ureter higher still and bringing it out as a high cutaneous ureterostomy as advocated by Lloyd et al. (1962). It is, of course, essential to consider this possibility in advance so that the stoma therapist can decide on the advisability of using a flank stoma.

Claman et al. (1979) reported ten cutaneous ureterostomies. Seven of the ten had normal-calibre ureters and of these two developed stenosis of the stoma which was corrected easily by simple stomal revision.

It is commonly said that care must be taken to avoid damaging the adventitia of the ureter but this is not enough to safeguard the blood supply. The longitudinal anastomotic vessels run a little distance away from the ureter and their preservation is essential. We have successfully used ureters of normal calibre in many patients.

The technique of Amin et al. (1977) seems very promising in enhancing the safety of using normal ureters. They have been using a method of terminal cutaneous ureterostomy that incorporates the advantages of loop ureterostomy. Their terminal loop cutaneous ureterostomy seems to eliminate stomal complications even in ureters of normal size. In their technique the ureter is brought out through the opening at the stomal site in the form of a loop with 2–3 cm of terminal ureter buried in the abdominal wall. The loop is prevented from retracting by suturing the fascia underneath and forming a protruding nipple. The exteriorised loop of the ureter is incised longitudinally at its apex and the edges of the ureterostomy are sutured to the skin edge producing a double barrelled stoma. The segment of ureter distal to the stoma is buried in the abdominal wall. Amin et al. have produced convincing evidence that this distal segment of the ureter develops a new blood supply from the surrounding tissues.

There is, however, little doubt that the blood supply is much less fragile when the ureter is dilated. Another factor that has to be taken into account is the size of the patient's abdomen. Relatively little ureter need to be mobilised in a very thin patient but in the obese subject the ureter might have to travel a considerable distance to reach the skin of the anterior abdominal wall. The more obese the patient, the greater the risk of ischaemic problems with cutaneous ureterostomy.

The best subject for urinary diversion by cutaneous ureterostomy in malignant disease is the relatively slim patient who has at least one ureter dilated to 1 cm or more. In such a patient it seems senseless to complicate matters and increase the risks by using a conduit to carry the urine from the ureter to the anterior abdominal wall, and, of course, the fact that a ureter is dilated is a contra-indication to uretero-colic anastomosis.

Diversion in the Radiated Patient

The difficulties that arise in urinary diversion in radiated patients are due to the fact that in treating a pelvic tumour such as carcinoma of the bladder or carcinoma of the cervix uteri with radical radiation it is impossible to avoid irradiating the ureters and bowel. Sophisticated modern techniques are designed to ensure the least possible radiation of structures other than the tumour and gross damage to neighbouring organs is nowadays rare.

Ureters and bowel subjected to fringe radiation will look normal and will remain perfectly healthy as long as they are not injured but it must be taken as axiomatic that radiated tissues heal poorly. The degree of healing deficit is directly proportional to the dose of radiation received by the tissues. In a review of 34 patients who underwent ureterosigmoidostomy after pelvic irradiation, O'Dea et al. (1977) found that the incidence of post-operative complications was greater after doses in excess of 5000 rads. They concluded that if the dose had been less than 5000 rads the incidence of complications after ureterosigmoidostomy was no greater than in patients who had not been radiated. As a general statement this is probably true but the one imponderable factor is the varition in individual response. This was highlighted in our experience (Walsh 1960) when a healthy man, aged 47, had radical cystectomy four months after radiotherapy to the bladder in which the maximum tumour dose was 4200 rads and the maximum skin dose 3800 rads. An ileal loop was used and intestinal continuity was restored with interrupted silk sutures. The patient died of septic complications five weeks after surgery. At autopsy the intestinal anastomosis appeared sound and the site was found only by tracing the black silk sutures which were still visible. These silk sutures were now carefully and gently removed and when this was done the anastomosis fell apart so that it was quite apparent that there had been little if any attempt at union between the ends of the intestine.

While the possibilities of radiation damage to the lower ureters, rectum and pelvic colon are obvious, it may not be so apparent to the inexperienced surgeon that loops of ileum may lie quite low in the pelvis and suffer similar radiation. A normal appearance of the bowel at surgery is no guarantee that it has not been subjected to significant radiation.

To minimise the risk of disintegration of anastomoses in radiated patients, the surgeon should assume that all tissues in the pelvis, including the lower ileum, may have been radiated to a significant degree. The ureters should be divided as high as possible above the pelvic brim. Indeed in operating for bladder cancer it is in any case advisable to remove a considerable length of ureter. It was reported by Wallace (1967) that one in every ten cystectomy specimens had tumour or in situ changes in the lower third of the ureter. In cases of bilharzia, lesions may well extend up the ureter, especially in the lower third and often to the middle third. We would agree with Wallace that any form of diversion may be designed so that the lower or even the middle third of the ureter can be excised if necessary. If uretero-colic anastomosis is the chosen method of diversion the lower iliac colon should be mobilised and displaced medially so that the anastomoses can be made above the pelvic brim. Similarly, if an isolated colo-rectal bladder is chosen the colon should be divided as high as possible. If a conduit is to be used it is obvious that one should use the high technique described by Wallace (1966). Terminal ileum should not be used for the conduit. At first sight it would seem that one should use jejunum but recent work has shown that electrolyte losses from a jejunal loop are so great that jejunum — certainly upper jejunum — should not be used. In most cases where a conduit is needed after radiation, the best material is probably transverse colon. It is fairly easy to make a conduit from a small centre section of transverse colon, based on the middle colic artery: the technique was reported in detail by Schmidt et al. (1975).

In performing any bowel anastomosis in the radiated patient, the sero-muscular layers should be approximated with interrupted sutures of unabsorbable material. Whether the ureters are led into intact colon or to a conduit, the entry should be tunnelled, not just to prevent reflux but also as an extra protection to the site of anastomosis.

If there is any significant degree of radiation proctitis, it is probably unwise to divert the ureters to the colon.

An interesting way of side-stepping the problems of urinary diversion in the radiated patient was reported by Mahoney et al. (1975). They described 47 patients with bladder carcinoma whose management was carried out in steps. The first step consisted of laparotomy staging and urinary diversion. Two weeks after this operation, radical radiation was begun and 6–8 weeks after completing radiotherapy, radical cystectomy was performed. There was only one death in the series and the authors attributed the low mortality rate to the staging of the operative procedures. The advisability of staging is discussed in a following section. A similar approach to that of Mahoney et al. was reported by Grimes et al. (1972).

Diversion in Advanced Malignant Disease

There are many patients with locally advanced pelvic carcinoma, perhaps untreated, perhaps already subjected to major surgery or radiotherapy or both, for whom the question may arise: Should the urine be diverted, and if so, how? The three main reasons for posing this question are:

1) To relieve the distress of very severe dysuria and frequency.
2) To allay the discomfort of a malignant vesico-vaginal fistula.
3) To treat renal failure caused by ureteric obstruction.

We should start by considering the first two situations, although they are relatively uncommon, because the answers are reasonably straightforward. Very severe dysuria and frequency are fortunately unusual in patients with bladder carcinoma and if they do occur it may be possible to keep the patient comfortable with an indwelling urethral catheter. Some such patients, however, are not made comfortable by a catheter and they may even be worse if the catheter is blocked frequently by slough. In such cases the patient is grateful for the relief afforded by urinary diversion.

In the case of malignant vesico-vaginal fistula the indication for diversion is even stronger. Many such women with advanced pelvic disease do not have extensive metastases and may be in good general condition with a life expectancy of a year or more. Even if the expected survival is only a matter of weeks there is no reason why these women should be left in the stinking misery of a continuous leak of infected urine.

In such cases the diversion must be as simple as possible: the patient does not want the burden of major surgery. This precludes the use of ileal or colonic conduits and also procedures involving major laparotomy such as diversion to the intact colon or isolated rectum — procedures which are, in any case, undesirable in such patients because of the very strong possibility of poor sphincter control of fluid in the bowel. The diversion must be complete. Hence, ureterostomy-in-situ (Walsh 1967) is not a good answer because urine may leak around the tube and down to the bladder. Nephrostomy has often been used in this situation but the diversion may not be complete and the surgery is considerable. Percutaneous nephrostomy under X-ray control is a simple procedure but here again the urinary diversion is incomplete.

The simplest answer to the problem and one that we have found very satisfactory is to bring one ureter out as a cutaneous ureterostomy and to ligature the other ureter. This was first suggested by Huggins and Scott (1945) who reported nine cases treated successfully in this way and they commented particularly on the absence of renal pain on the side in which the ureter was tied. They reported a further two patients who had to have nephrectomy for pyonephrosis after ligature of the ureter. The same procedure was used by Young and Aledia (1966) on 19 patients but five required secondary nephrectomy. Our experience has been more fortunate. in the past 26 years we have used this technique in 22 patients and in only one was there any problem due to ligature of the ureter: this patient developed acute infected hydronephrosis and the kidney had to be removed.

The more dilated ureter should be chosen for the diversion, provided that renal function on that side is adequate. The technique is essentially the Lapides (1962) mark I technique. The ureter is approached extra-peritoneally through a small gridiron incision as low as possible in the appropriate iliac fossa. The ureter is divided no lower than the point at which it crosses the bifurcation of the iliac vessels and it is brought up in a smooth curve to the point on the abdomen previously marked by the stoma therapist. The end of the ureter is slit and a single skin flap is turned down in to this slit. It is wise to leave a catheter in the ureter for a few days. This catheter is passed up to the renal pelvis and is cut off about 1 cm distal to the stoma. A small sterile pin is placed in the end of the catheter to prevent it falling in and the appliance can be fitted over this immediately. The ureter on the other side is ligatured through a similar approach. Only a small gridiron incision is necessary to expose the ureter but it is important to be certain of identification: in one case in our series the ovarian vein was ligatured by mistake instead of the ureter. We use two ligatures of heavy silk. A thick ligature material is less likely to cut through the ureter.

The third possible indication for diversion, to relieve ureteric obstruction causing renal failure, is the one that leads to most heart searching. It is clearly bad medicine to subject a patient to surgery in order to exchange death from uremia this week for a painful and miserable end a very few weeks later. On the other hand, if there is any possibility of effective therapy for the tumour and there is a possibility of good quality survival for a year or two, the obstruction should be relieved (Chisholm and Shackman 1968). I would agree with Fallon et al. (1980) that there is little doubt that diversion should be strongly considered where the malignant disease was previously undiagnosed and therefore untreated.

The patient's own feelings should be respected above all else. We must recognise that it may be very important to a patient to prolong his life for even a short time for some financial or personal reason.

A significant factor in this very difficult decision is the tissue or origin of the tumour. It is clear from the work of Fallon et al. (1980) and from the studies of Brin et al. (1975), of Khan and Utz (1975) and of Van Dyke and Van Nagell (1975) that patients whose primary lesion is in the prostate or uterine cervix do much better than any others. The study by Khan and Utz makes the important point that there is a much better survival among patients with prostate carcinoma who have not been treated with hormones previously and they believe that one is almost obliged to treat aggressively such patients in whom the malignant prostate may respond to hormone manipulation, unless there is extensive metastatic diseases causing serious pain. Very occasionally, in a patient with locally extensive carcinoma of the prostate only, the obstruction to both ureters can be simply relieved by uretero-neo-cystomy — the ureters being simply re-implanted into the dome of the bladder.

Our own experience is entirely in agreement with the work of the authors quoted above. It is very rarely wise to advise diversion in the patient with transitional cell carcinoma of the bladder or colorectal carcinoma where survival rates and quality of life are dismal.

There is a special case for diversion in the patient whose ureters are obstructed by malignant retro-peritoneal lymphoma. Indeed, many patients with retro-peritoneal malignant disease first present with obstruction of the abdominal ureters and in such patients the obstruction must be relieved to allow time to establish the diagnosis and the possibilities of treatment. By far the best method of relieving the obstruction in this situation is the use of the silicone rubber stent devised by Gibbons et al. (1974). In the very few cases where it is not possible to place a Gibbons stent the procedure of choice is percutaneous nephrostomy or ureterostomy-in-situ.

A very similar problem is presented by ureteric obstruction from metastatic breast cancer. Grabstald and Kaufman (1969) described 24 such cases seen between 1960 and 1967 in the Memorial Hospital, New York. The Gibbons stent would seem an ideal solution in this situation if the patient is a young woman who has not had hormone therapy. We would agree with Holden et al. (1979) that a similar patient in an older age group who has had failed hormonal therapy, radiotherapy and chemo-therapy and who is now out of control would be better left alone.

It will seldom be possible to pass a Gibbons stent in cases where the ureter is obstructed by carcinoma of the prostate or cervix. The method of diversion most commonly used in such cases is nephrostomy. Open surgical nephrostomy is, however, an unnecessarily large procedure. Percutaneous nephrostomy under local analgesia is much better but often not satisfactory for prolonged drainage. Probably the best method of diversion in these cases is ureterostomy-in-situ.

Nephrostomy

There is a curious divergence in practice on the two sides of the Atlantic. As a method of urinary diversion in patients with malignant disease, nephrostomy is quite common in the United States (Fallon et al. 1980) but it is relatively little used in Great Britain or in Ireland. As an open surgical procedure, nephrostomy is a major undertaking. In this regard the recent development by radiologists of techniques of percutaneous intubation of the kidney under X-ray control is a considerable step forward. One of the many problems with nephrostomy is that if it is maintained for any length of time infection can be a serious complication and may lead to secondary haemorrhage. Another disadvantage is that it is often difficult to change a nephro-stomy tube. Tresidder (1957) devised an ingenious technique to solve the latter problem (Fig. 4.4). The Tresidder U-tube certainly gets over the problem of changing tubes but it does require full exposure of the kidney. Another problem is that the nephrostomy tube is liable to emerge in the flank where it is awkward and uncomfortable.

Ureterostomy-in-situ

This technique was largely abandoned and forgotten when many ureters were seriously damaged by the old red rubber catheters. The operation was reinstated (Walsh 1967) with the development of biologically inert plastic materials (Fig. 4.5). The author emphasised that the catheter should be brought out through a stab wound in the anterior abdominal wall as low as possible so that it runs in a gentle curve to the ureter. The catheter should be lying parallel with the ureter at its point of entry into the ureter. Care is taken to avoid damage to the peritoneum or to the external iliac artery. A longitudinal ureterostomy is made at least twice the diameter of the catheter and after inserting the catheter the ureteric incision should not be sutured around it.

Attention to these technical details allows the catheter to be changed two to three weeks later and thereafter every two weeks for as long as it is necessary to maintain

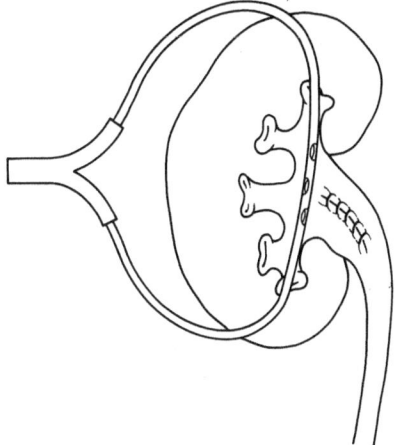

Fig.4.4. Loop nephrostomy (Tresidder).

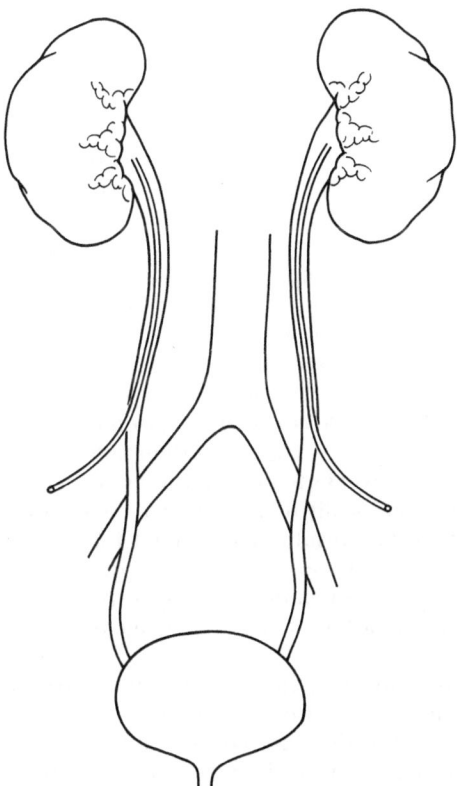

Fig.4.5. Ureterostomy-in-situ (Walsh).

the diversion. Even when ureterostomy-in-situ has been maintained for many months, urinary infection has not been a problem as occurs with prolonged nephrostomy drainage. The operation is quick and simple to perform and the tube emerges at a point that is easy to manage.

The catheter used is either a PVC infant feeding tube or a Foley catheter and should be only 10F or 12F and not an 18FG catheter as originally recommended in 1967. A large catheter can cause ischaemic pressure necrosis at the pelvic-ureteric junction producing a secondary stricture.

Ureterostomy-in-situ is rarely used as a method of permanent diversion and then only as a palliative procedure in terminal cancer patients distressed by very severe urinary tract symptoms. In such cases the ureters should be ligated in continuity below the point of entry of the catheters so that the bladder will be completely defunctioned.

Dialysis

This is very rarely indicated in a patient with renal failure caused by malignant ureteric obstruction. If anything is to be done at all, the sooner the urine is diverted the better. About the only indication for dialysis in such patients is a degree of acidosis that would make anaesthesia dangerous. If the blood bicarbonate is below 12 mmol/l or if the potassium is dangerously high a single short haemodialysis or a few hours peritoneal dialysis should be all that is needed to correct the biochemical disorder sufficiently to make anaesthesia reasonably safe.

Staging of Diversion and Cancer Surgery

The great majority of urologists treating bladder cancer by cystectomy perform the urinary diversion at the same time. There is undoubtedly pressure to carry out all the surgery in one stage in countries where hospital costs are very high but in our view there is an overriding factor of increased safety in very poor risk patients when the procedures are staged. In the earlier section in this chapter 'Diversion in the radiated patient', reference has already been made to the reports of Mahoney et al. (1975) and of Grimes et al. (1972). In personal discussion in 1980, the senior author of the latter paper, Glenn, explained that one reason for embarking on two-stage diversion-cystectomy was the discovery that the surgically related mortality in patients under-going a one-stage procedure had been over 15%. Accordingly, they embarked on a series of 50 consecutive staged patients, doing the diversion first, then radiating, then performing the cystectomy anywhere from two weeks to two months later. In the first 50 patients treated in this way there were no surgically related deaths. Glenn felt that staging was not the only factor in the improved results. He thought the quality of surgery was improving and that support facilities were better. They then began to select patients for staging. If the patient was fragile and a poor operative risk they would elect a two-stage approach, but now in most patients a one-stage procedure is used.

We would agree very strongly with this attitude. In the relatively fit patient a single-stage procedure is probably best. However, there is no doubt in our minds that in the very old or very debilitated patient the risks are considerably reduced by staging the surgery. Our reasoning is that when the urine is diverted to a conduit or to the colon, there is inevitably some oedema at the site of anastomosis and this may embarrass kidney function in the vital first few days when the kidneys have to deal with a huge metabolic load if radical pelvic surgery is performed at the same time.

Our method of staging differs from that described above. In such elderly, poor risk, patients we prefer, where possible, to use the isolated recto-sigmoid and then we proceed exactly as described by Pyrah (1963). At the first stage, through a mid-line abdominal incision, laparotomy is performed to determine the extent of the tumour and the degree, if any, of lymph node spread. Then the sigmoid colon is divided as high as possible and a terminal left iliac colostomy is fashioned. The left ureter is now isolated, divided and, in most cases, passed through a small opening in the base of the meso-sigmoid. The ureter is then implanted into the upper part of the recto-sigmoid bladder. Some weeks later, when it is certain that the transplanted ureter is functioning well, with a good output of rectal urine in a well patient with no fistula, the abdomen is reopened through the same midline incision, the bladder is removed and the divided right ureter is anastomosed to the recto-sigmoid bladder.

The advantage of this method of staging is that one can be sure that one kidney is, so to speak, back in action and functioning well with free drainage into the recto-sigmoid when the major extirpative surgery is undertaken. A disadvantage of proceeding in this fashion is that it makes it more difficult to carry our radical clearance of the lymph nodes with the cystectomy but we are not convinced that this is a serious objection in the type of patient under consideration.

We reported the use of this two-stage procedure in 17 patients aged 75 or over, the oldest being 83 (Walsh 1977). There was no mortality and minimum morbidity. Since then we have used the staged procedure in two more patients: in one of these, a man aged 84, the urine was diverted to the intact colon and in this patient the right ureter was implanted at the first stage. Three weeks later the bladder was removed and the left ureter implanted. Both patients had an uneventful recovery.

Staging in this way is not practical with conduit diversion in which both ureters will have to be diverted at the first stage. Where cutaneous ureterostomy is the chosen technique, staging is not indicated.

Technical Considerations in Reducing Surgical Mortality

There is a great variation from centre to centre in the mortality and mordibity of urinary diversion for malignant disease. Even in the best series, there is a recurrent theme of infection, paralytic ileus and dehiscence of abdominal wounds.

Paralytic ileus is much less common now than 25 years ago and much of the credit for this is due to advances in anaesthetic techniques, the use of antibiotics and early mobilisation of the patient after surgery. Very important factors in preventing this complication include gentle handling of bowel and mesenteries and also prevention of sepsis.

Infection is always a risk when the bowel is open, particularly the large bowel. Matheson and Valerio (1980) have pointed out that the hazards of large bowel surgery can usually be avoided by a good antibiotic lavage for extant or potential peritoneal and wound contamination. It is now quite clear that the most important single factor in bowel preparation is complete mechanical cleansing. In this context an important advance in recent times has been the introduction of whole-gut irrigation (Hewitt et al. 1973). As described by these authors, the irrigant solution contains 6.14 g sodium chloride, 0.75 g potassium chloride, and 2.94 g sodium bicarbonate in each litre. If glucose is added there is increased absorption of sodium and water from the gut: glucose should not be used. Some 10–12 litres of irrigating fluid are run into the stomach through an oro-gastric or naso-gastric tube while the patient sits on a commode or on a 'cholera couch'. Metronidazole 1.6 g and neomycin sulphate 20 g are added to the irrigation fluid, which is run in until the fluid emerging from the bowel has been clear for about 1 hour. The total irrigation time is usually 2–3 hours.

Patients who have experienced both this technique and the standard routine of cathartics and enemas find whole-gut irrigation less tiring and less distasteful. For patient acceptability, it is very important to prevent nausea and this is a matter of careful regulation of rate of flow of the irrigating fluid. As soon as there is the slightest hint of nausea the flow should be stopped briefly until the sensation passes and the flow is restarted at a slightly lower rate.

The use of metronidazole to deal with Bacteroides is another important recent advance. In addition, Matheson and Valerio recommend lavage of the peritoneal cavity with 500 ml of warm saline containing 500 mg tetracycline and also a single peroperative intravenous dose of 500 mg tetracycline.

There is widespread agreement now that bowel anastomoses should be made with a single layer of interrupted non-absorbable, sero-muscular sutures. Silk as a suture material has been replaced in many centres by braided polyamide.

Debilitated patients with malignant disease are notoriously liable to wound dehiscence. The surgeon should not overlook the value of parenteral nutrition in many of these patients. The actual dehiscence is not normally due to breakdown of suture material but is caused by the stitches cutting out of the tissue of the abdominal wall. This complication can be virtually eliminated by the use of a continuous far and near stitch of unabsorbable monofilament material such as prolene. This stitch is laid in loosely in a figure-of-eight with the far component passing at least 3 cm from the wound edge, through all layers of the abdominal wall (except skin). The near component of the stitch ensures accurate approximation of the edges of the external oblique aponeurosis. The stitch must be laid in and not pulled tight.

Envoi

The whole question of diversion in the patient with malignant disease calls for the most careful and delicate judgement. This is especially obvious in the case of bladder cancer where the survival and the quality of survival of the patient depend on the good judgement of the urologist who makes the diagnosis. There is little doubt that many patients with extensive papillary carcinoma are subjected unnecessarily to the hazards of cystectomy when in fact they could be managed by transurethral resection. On the other hand, patients with solid bladder tumours must be treated radically immediately but, here again, there can be a difficult problem of judgement between the merits of radiotherapy and radical surgery in a particular case.

If diversion is unavoidable, it is our hope that the urologist will have all the possible techniques at his command so that he can make the best choice for each individual patient.

References

Amin M, Clark R, Howerton LW, Lich R Jr (1977) Terminal loop cutaneous ureterostomy: An experimental study and its clinical application. J Urol 118: 383–385

Blackard CE, Nicolaidis AN, Johnston JD (1973) Modified loop cutaneous ureterostomy. J Urol 110: 291–293

Brin EN, Schiff M Jr, Weiss RM (1975) Palliative urinary diversion for pelvic malignancy. J Urol 113: 619–622

Castro JE, Ram MD (1970) Electrolyte imbalance following ileal urinary diversion. Br J Urol 42: 29–32

Chisholm GD (1977) Die Nierenfunktion nach Harnableitung. In: Zingg E, Tscholl R (eds) Die supravesikale Harnableitung. Huber, Bern, pp 88–94

Chisholm GD, Shackman R (1968) Malignant obstructive uraemia. Br J Urol 40: 720–726

Claman M, Schapiro AE, Orecklin JR (1979) Cutaneous ureterostomy, the preferred diversion of the solitary functioning kidney. Br J Urol 51: 352–356

Clark PB (1979) End-to-end ureteroileal anastomosis for ileal conduits. Br J Urol 51: 105–109

Cordonnier JJ (1949) Ureterosigmoid anastomosis. Surg Gynecol Obstet 88: 441–446

Culp DA, Flocks RH (1966) The diversion of urine by the Heitz-Boyer procedure. J Urol 95: 334–343

Daniel O, Ram RS (1965) The value of sigmoid myotomy in reducing bowel pressure and thus averting renal damage following uretero-colic anastomosis. Br J Urol 37: 654–659

Elder DD, Moisey CU, Rees RWM (1979) A long-term follow-up of the colonic conduit operation in children. Br J Urol 51: 462–465

Ensor RD, Atwill WH, Secrest AJ, Leitner WA, Glenn JF (1970) The modified Gersuny procedure for urinary diversion. J Urol 104: 93–97

Fallon B, Olney L, Culp DA (1980) Nephrostomy in cancer patients: to do or not to do? Br J Urol 52: 237–242

Gersuny R (1898) Cited by Foges: Officielles protokll der K K gesellschaft der aerzte in Wien. Wien Klin Wochenschr 11: 990

Ghoneim MA, Ashamallah A (1974) Further experience with the rectosigmoid bladder. Br J Urol 46: 511–519

Ghoneim MA, Shehab-El-Din AB, Ashamallah AK and Gaballah MA (1981) Evolution of Rectal Bladder as Method of Urinary Diversion. J Urol 126: 737–740

Gibbons RP, Mason JT, Correa RJ Jr (1974) Experience with indwelling silicone rubber ureteral catheters. J Urol 111: 594–599

Goodwin WE, Harris AP, Kaufman JJ, Beal JM (1953) Open, transcolonic uretero-intestinal anastomosis: A new approach. Surg Gynecol Obstet 97: 282–295

Grabstald H, Kaufman R (1969) Hydronephrosis secondary to ureteral obstruction by metastatic breast cancer. J Urol 102: 569–576

Grimes JH, Hart JM, Glenn JF, Anderson EE (1972) Staged approach to invasive vesical malignancy. J Urol 108: 872–874

Hammer E (1929) Cancer du colon sigmoîde dix ans après implantation des uretères d'une vessie exstrophiée. J Urol 28: 260–263

Hawtrey CE, Boatman DL, Brown RG, Schmidt JD (1974) Clinical experience with loop nephrostomy for urinary diversion. J Urol 112: 36–41

Heitz-Boyer M, Hovelacque A (1912) Création d'une nouvelle vessie et un nouvel urètre. J Urol 1: 237–258

Hewitt J, Reeve J, Rigby J, Cox AG (1973) Whole-gut irrigation in preparation for large bowel surgery. Lancet II: 337–340

Hohenfellner R (1977) Ureterosigmoidostomy. In: Eckstein HB, Hohenfellner R, Williams DI (eds) Surgical pediatric urology. Thieme, Stuttgart, p 347

Holden S, McPhee M, Grabstald H (1979) The rationale of urinary diversion in cancer patients. J Urol 121: 19–21

Huggins C, Scott WW (1945) Cutaneous ureterostomy with contralateral ureteral ligation. J Urol 53: 325–338

Jacobs A (1953) Transplantation of the ureters — indications and methods. In: Riches EW (ed) Modern trends in urology. Butterworth, London, pp 179–190

Khan AU, Utz DC (1975) Clinical management of carcinoma of prostate associated with bilateral ureteral obstruction. J Urol 113: 816–819

Lapides J (1962) Butterfly cutaneous ureterostomy. J Urol 88: 735–739

Leadbetter WF (1951) Consideration of problems incident to the performance of uretero-enterostomy: Report of a technique. J Urol 65: 818–830

Lee SW, Russel J, Avioli LV (1977) 25 hydroxycholecalciferol to 1,25-dihydroxycholecalciferol conversion impaired by systemic metabolic acidosis. Science 195: 994–996

Lloyd FA, Cottrell TLC, Cross RR, Calams J (1962) High cutaneous ureterostomy. J Urol 88: 740–745

Mahoney EM, Weber ET, Harrison JH (1975) Post-diversion pre-cystectomy irradiation for carcinoma of the bladder. J Urol 114: 46–49

Matheson NA, Valerio D (1980) Large bowel surgery, 1979: Self-assessment. Br Med J ii: 719–721

Milroy MD, Thompson IM, Depauw AP, Ross GR Jr (1978) Permanent cutaneous ureterostomy: 18 years of experience. J Urol 120: 682–684

Mogg RA (1965) The treatment of neurogenic urinary incontinence using the colonic conduit. Br J Urol 37: 681–686

Nesbit RM (1949) Ureterosigmoid anastomosis by direct elliptical connection: A preliminary report. J Urol 61: 728–734

O'Dea MJ, Barrett DM, Segura JW (1977) Ureterosigmoidostomy after pelvic irradiation. J Urol 118: 386–387

Pyrah LN (1963) The rectosigmoid bladder as a method of urinary diversion. J Urol 90: 189–192

Schmidt JD, Hawtrey CE, Flocks RH, Culp DA (1973) Complications, results and problems of ileal conduit diversions. J Urol 109: 210–216

Schmidt JD, Hawtrey CE, Buchsbaum HJ (1975) Transverse colon conduit: A preferred method of urinary diversion for radiation-treated pelvic malignancies. J Urol 113: 308–313

Shehab El Din (1979) Evolution of the rectal bladder as a method for urinary diversion. Thesis for Master of Urology, Mansoura, Egypt

Spence HM, Hoffman WW, Fosmire GP (1979) Tumour of the colon as a late complication of uretero-sigmoidostomy for exstrophy of the bladder. Br J Urol 51: 466–470

Stamey TA (1956) The pathogenesis and implications of the electrolyte imbalance in uretero-sigmoidostomy. Surg Gynecol Obstet 103: 736–???

Stewart M, Hill MJ, Pugh RCB, Williams JP (1981) The role of N-nitrosamine in carcinogenesis at the uretero-colic anastomosis. Br J Urol 53: 115–118

Straffon RA, Kyle K, Corvalan J (1970) Techniques of cutaneous ureterostomy and results in 51 patients. J Urol 103: 138–146

Thompson IM, Ross G Jr (1963) Experiences with a new technique for supravesical urinary diversion. J Urol 90: 691–695

Tresidder GC (1957) Nephrostomy. Br J Urol 29: 130–134

Turner-Warwick RT (1976) Three-option ureterosigmoidostomy. In: Blandy J (ed) Urology. Blackwell, Oxford, p 1107

Van Dyke AH, Van Nagell JR Jr (1975) The prognostic significance of ureteral obstruction in patients with recurrent carcinoma of the cervix uteri. Surg Gynecol Obstet 141: 371–373

Vereecken RL, Dewaele HM, Kerremans R, Penninckx F, Proesmans W (1980) Pre-operative and post-operative evaluation of the rectal bladder. Br J Urol 52: 285–289

Wallace DM (1966) Ureteric diversion using a conduit: A simplified technique. Br J Urol 38: 522–527

Wallace DM (1967) Ileal conduit. Br J Urol 39: 681–686

Walsh A (1960) Hazards of bladder surgery following irradiation. J Urol 84: 627–629

Walsh A (1967) Ureterostomy in situ. Br J Urol 39: 744–745

Walsh A (1977) Die Rektosigmoidblase nach Mauclaire. In: Zingg E, Tscholl R (eds) Die supravesikale Harnableitung. Huber, Bern, p 245–246

Williams RE, Davenport TJ, Burkinshaw L, Hughes D (1967) Changes in whole body potassium associated with uretero-intestinal anastomoses. Br J Urol 39: 676–680

Winterborn MH, Mace PJ, Heath DA, White RHR (1978) Impairment of renal function in patients on 1α-hydroxycholecalciferol. Lancet II: 150–151

Young JD Jr, Aledia FT (1966) Further observations on flank ureterostomy and cutaneous trans-ureteroureterostomy. J Urol 95: 327–333

Zincke H, Segura JW (1975) Ureterosigmoidostomy: Critical review of 173 cases. J Urol 113: 324–327

Chapter 5
Stoma Care

Auriol L. Lawson

Introduction

The concept of radical and amputative surgery could be carried to such a stage that
what was left with the patient became a consideration of equal importance to that
which was removed. It seemed that if we could not leave a patient in a physiological
state compatible with a comfortable existence, we were not morally justified in doing
some of the extensive procedures. (Bricker 1950)

Bricker was aware that traumatic and disfiguring surgery, no matter how essential,
should allow the patient to return to a normal life, relatively unaffected by that surgery.
Thirty years later, there are still many surgeons and nurses who do not appreciate the
emotional and psychological impact of stoma surgery, or the importance of adequate
preoperative preparation. The acceptance of an abdominal stoma by the patient and
his family is often dependent upon the amount of time and consideration given to
patient counselling, and the assurance that the operation will only be of benefit to them
(Fig. 5.1). There is a growing awareness among medical and nursing personnel that
every potential stoma patient has their individual needs and considerations; and a
recognition that management can be improved with the provision of a nurse specialist
in this field. The appointment of such a Clinical Nurse Specialist in Stoma Care is
becoming accepted in many areas of the British Isles, and acting in an advisory capacity
she has become responsible for the emotional well-being of her patients, providing a
valuable source of information for them and their families. Stoma care nurses, working
closely with a surgical team are able to recognise and treat specific problems associated
with abdominal stomas. Close follow-up of every patient in specially formed stoma
clinics has helped to create high standards of care, and the prevention and early
detection of long-term complications. Stoma nurses must have an amicable and ready
access to patients both in the hospital wards and on a long-term follow-up domiciliary
service to the patient's home.

Training and Numbers of Stoma Nurses

Enterostomal therapy is now established on an international basis and there are annual
meetings of the World Council of Enterostomal Therapists involving stoma nurses
from many continents of the world. Physicians and surgeons, from many different

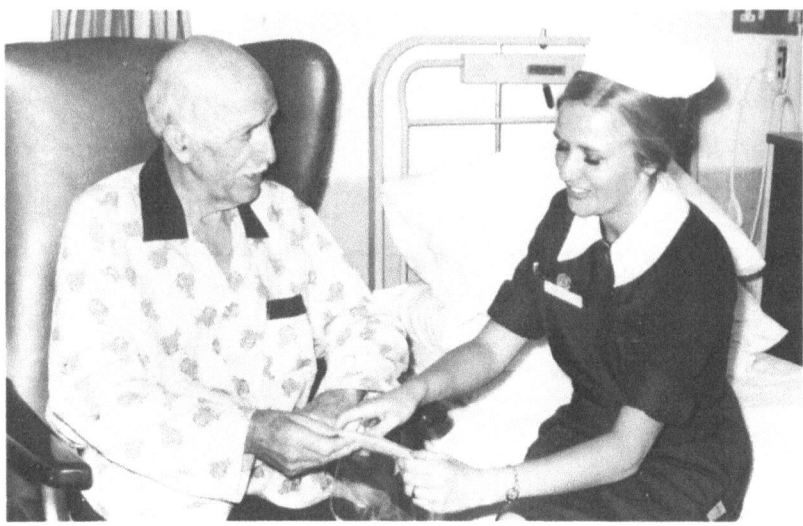

Fig.5.1. Patient counselling.

countries, with known interests and expertise in the treatment of stoma patients are invited to contribute at these meetings. A book on Enterostomal Therapy (May 1977) gives a comprehensive reference guide for the successful care of ostomy patients including a glossary of terms, diagrams and lists of training schools accredited by the International Association for Enterostomal Therapy.

There are now approximately 120 stoma nurses working in various centres throughout the British Isles. Such nurses may be hospital- or community-based, or ideally be part-funded by both hospital and community. As members of the nursing team they are normally funded from the nursing budget, despite their working closely with doctors in hospital and the community. The private sector does not employ stoma care nurses, but private patients may be referred to a National Health Service-funded nurse by their respective surgeons and a fee charged for these services. The stoma nurse must carry out this work outside of normal working hours.

The manufacturers of ostomy equipment employ qualified nurses as their representatives to sell their products, and act as a source of advice and information for stoma patients. Appliance fitters who are employed by surgical appliance firms do not necessarily hold a nursing qualification, but some are known as stomatherapists, and may even be ostomists themselves. State Registered Nurses wishing to specialise in stoma care may be accepted for training on to a course recognised by the Joint Board of Clinical Nursing Studies, of which there are four at present (London, Stockton, Manchester, and Birmingham). Each nurse must have at least 2 years' postgraduate experience, preferably at Ward Sister level and British nurses should be seconded to the course by their employing authority.

The number of stoma care nurses employed in the Health Service bears no relation to the numbers required nationally to provide an adequate service; many Health Authorities are still without any such nurses, whereas others employ more than one.

The workload of stoma nurses varies considerably from area to area, and it has proved almost impossible to arrive at a national figure of the number of nurses required. It would be necessary to take into account the number of hospitals and health centres each nurse had to cover, the distance between them, and the size of the geographical area. More home visits would be required for the less mobile elderly patients, therefore the age of the local population must also be considered.

Specialist units such as Radiotherapy and Gastro-Enterology where patients may be referred, must also be taken into account, as the distance between them may extend from one area health authority into another.

Number of Patients with Abdominal Stomas

The number of patients with permanent abdominal stomas in one particular area is often the deciding factor which determines the need for a clinical nurse specialist in stoma care. The precise number of permanent stomas in Great Britain is not known with any degree of accuracy, but the figures most often quoted are those resulting from a survey undertaken by Talbot in 1975 (Table 5.1). The total number of temporary stomas is unknown.

Table 5.1. Annual and total numbers of permanent stomas in Great Britain (Talbot 1975)

Permanent stomas	Annually	Total in Great Britain
Colostomy	3000	100000
Ileostomy	1000	17500
Ileal conduit	450	9000
	4450	126500

Jones et al. (1980), in a survey undertaken at the Royal Marsden Hospital in London, indicate that Talbot's figures for new ileal conduits are too low. Completed questionnaires from members of the British Association of Urological Surgeons gave a total figure of 402 new ileal conduits between 1976 and 1977, and 387 between 1977 and 1978. Only 57 members of the British Association of Urological Surgeons completed the questionnaire out of a total of 151 sent out, showing that even this low proportion of urologists approaches Talbot's figures.

The assurance of a satisfactory and efficient stoma care service is dependent upon the provision of an adequate back-up service by the employing authority. Clerical and secretarial help are vital to a stoma nurse if she is to function independently and provide a continuation of care from hospital to community. Some form of transportation is essential for stoma nurses who cover large distances between hospitals and in the community.

Ideally, the nurse should be based within easy access of hospital wards and out-patient departments, and provision made for suitable consulting facilities. The use of a telephone and bleep are essential for stoma nurses based in hospital who are constantly moving between wards and departments, to facilitate contact with patient services in the community such as the family practitioner, health visitor, social services department, local pharmacists, district nurses and local authorities.

Storage and Ordering of Ostomy Equipment

Many stoma nurses are responsible for the storage and ordering of ostomy equipment for use in the hospital and clinics, hence the need for adequate storage space. Considerable expense and wastage can be prevented, and thoughtless ordering of unnecessary and obsolete equipment avoided. The evaluation and standardisation of ostomy equipment is largely the responsibility of the stoma nurse who is in an ideal position to select patients willing to test proposed additions to the appliance market. This enables manufacturers to produce equipment which has been tried and accepted by ostomists, and to make modifications wherever necessary. The standardisation of equipment for use postoperatively on surgical units, reduces wastage and prevents confusion amongst nursing staff and patients.

In recent years the management of urinary diversion stomas has changed considerably. This is in part due to the advent of the lightweight disposable appliance, which, in comparison to its forerunner, the bulky rubber variety, requires the minimum of effort to apply and maintain. Bags are supplied in different sizes to cover all age groups and variable social requirements and many bags have non-return valves to avoid reflux of urine when in the supine position. Close supervision of the urostomy patient helps prevent complications which in the past may have required long spells in hospital. The training of each patient to become independent and self confident in the management of their urostomy must take place before discharge from hospital.

Stoma Site

Careful planning of the stoma site preoperatively reduces the incidence of skin excoriation caused by leakage of urine from badly sited stomas (Fig. 5.2). In many hospitals stoma siting is as much the responsibility of the stoma nurse as of the surgeon. Old scars, natural creases, the waistline, umbilicus and underlying bones are sites of potential leakage to be avoided if possible (Fig. 5.3). Disabilities such as missing limbs, failing eyesight and diminished hand and finger movements must be given thoughtful consideration before urinary diversion is contemplated (Fig. 5.4). Thought must be given to the lifestyle of each patient; his work, pastimes and hobbies. Obese patients with large abdomens require particular attention when planning the site of the proposed stoma. It is always useful to examine the abdomen with the patient standing upright, sitting and recumbent. In these patients, the site often needs to be marked slightly higher than usual to allow clear visibility and easy access for the patient when managing the stoma independently.

Siting of the stoma may be particularly difficult in patients with multiple sclerosis, paraplegia or spina bifida, who spend long periods in wheelchairs. It is important to ensure that the stoma is placed in a position which is comfortable and sufficiently flat to prevent leakage from the appliance (Fig. 5.5). The patient will often benefit from a preoperative trial wearing of an urostomy bag containing some water to simulate the weight of urine collecting in the bag.

Complications of Stomas

Leakage

The basic principles of stoma care apply equally to all abdominal stomas, but there are particular problems associated with urostomies. Patients may often deal with minor leakage and skin problems themselves, but should know when to seek professional help. Advising patients of the possibility and causes of skin irritation and leakage

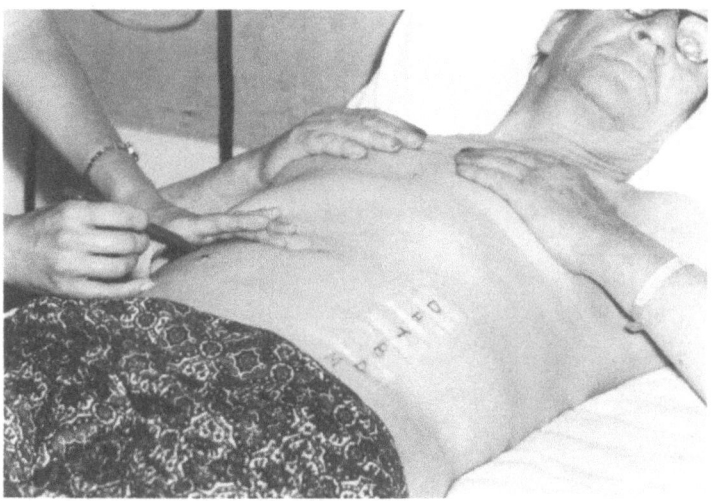

Fig.5.2. Planning stoma site—patient recumbent.

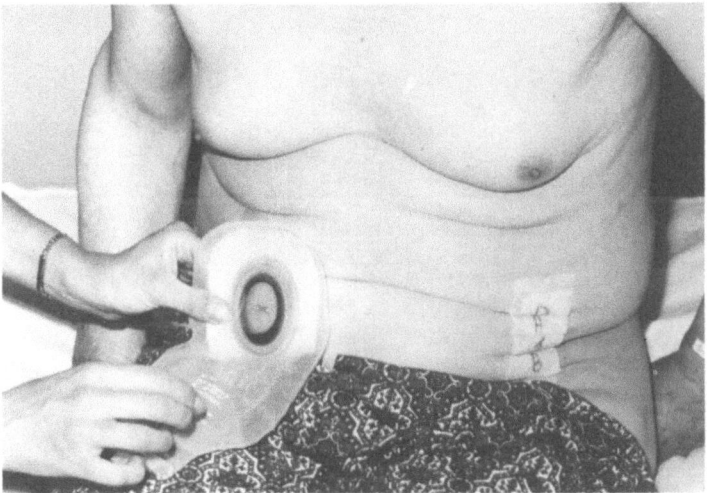

Fig.5.3. Planning stoma site, avoiding creases and waistline, etc.

following urinary diversion is an essential part of their 'training programme' prior to discharge from hospital.

Despite an increasing awareness of the importance of stoma siting, badly sited stomas remain a common cause of leakage which can give rise to sore skin, which in turn causes difficulty in adhesion of the appliance faceplate. This results in further leakage and so a vicious circle is established, causing anxiety to the patient.

Careful preparation of the peristomal skin, and centralisation of the stoma, when applying a urostomy appliance is essential if leakage is to be prevented. Care must be taken to ensure that the peristomal skin is thoroughly dry and that the adhesive faceplace of the appliance is smooth and free from wrinkles and creases. Frequent measuring of the stoma for shrinkage prevents problems caused by a gasket which is

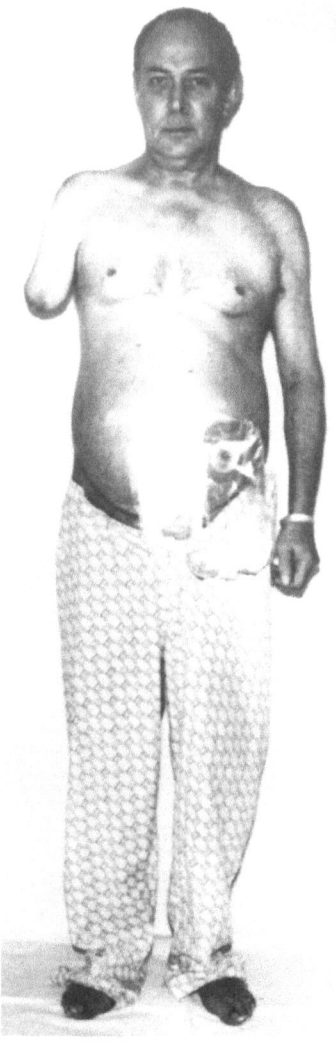

Fig.5.4. Patient disabilities.

either too large or too small. Manufacturing faults in equipment due to automated mass production has led many patients to anticipate leakage from faulty seams and tap welds on some modern appliances, so that they should carefully examine disposable pouches before use. Irate nurses, pharmacists, surgical appliance suppliers, and above all, patients, are a constant reminder to manufacturers of ostomy equipment that their products are not always up to standard and that improvements are often necessary.

Disposable appliances are designed to be applied directly to the skin by means of an adhesive faceplate. The application of a skin barrier (e.g. Karaya, Stomahesive, Reliaseal) is sometimes required to provide additional adhesion around the stoma by forming a watertight seal. Skin barriers may also be used to treat and prevent allergic reactions from adhesive faceplates. Many skin barriers remain intact for several days even though they are used as an integral part of a urostomy appliance. Leakage may occur when the skin barrier has dissolved, usually after 3–4 days, and will require renewal. A quick and easy method of applying a skin barrier is to attach it to the appliance faceplate first and then apply them both as a one-piece unit.

Flush ureterostomy and retracted ileal conduit stomas often lead to seepage of urine from beneath the appliance faceplate. Peristomal dermatitis, infection and discomfort quickly ensue if left untreated (Fig. 5.6). Sometimes the stoma may appear to have retracted if the patient has an excessive weight gain after operation, hence the 'sinking stoma'. Retraction may be corrected by applying pressure to the peristomal area by means of a rigid faceplate and a belt, which will help to project the stoma. If this is not satisfactory, weight reduction or surgical revision may be necessary. Cutaneous ureterostomies which are nearly always flush require close supervision to ensure that problems with leakage are prevented.

The optimum length of the ileal conduit stoma has been the subject of controversy. Patients with flush urinary stomas have more problems with leakage, periostomal dermatitis and infection than those with protruding stomas (Jeter 1976). Ideally, urinary stomas should protrude from the surface of the skin by 2–3 cm so that the urine is conveyed directly into the collecting apparatus.

Difficulties are also encountered by patients when attempting to centralise the appliance faceplate over a flush stoma; this can be overcome by the use of a mirror, or centralising tube. Urinary stomas which exceed 5 cm are not always satisfactory. Apart from the risk of impairment to the blood supply, some patients, especially women, find a long stoma psychologically unacceptable and repulsive.

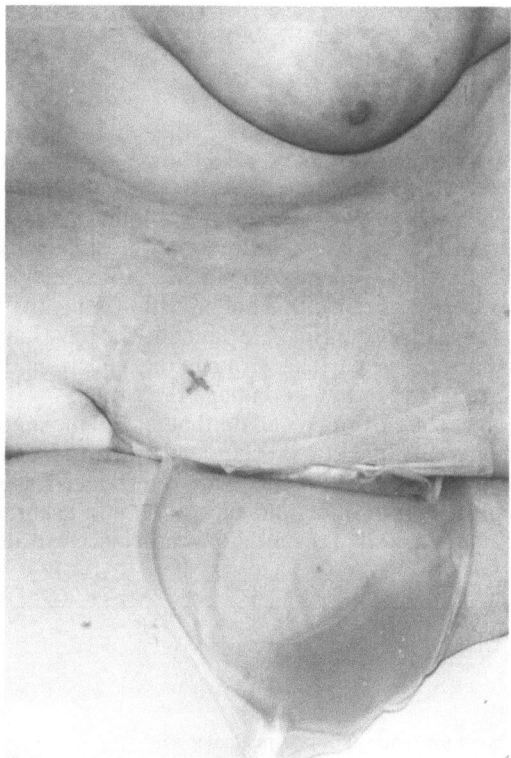

Fig.5.5. Wheelchair-bound patient—selecting alternative site.

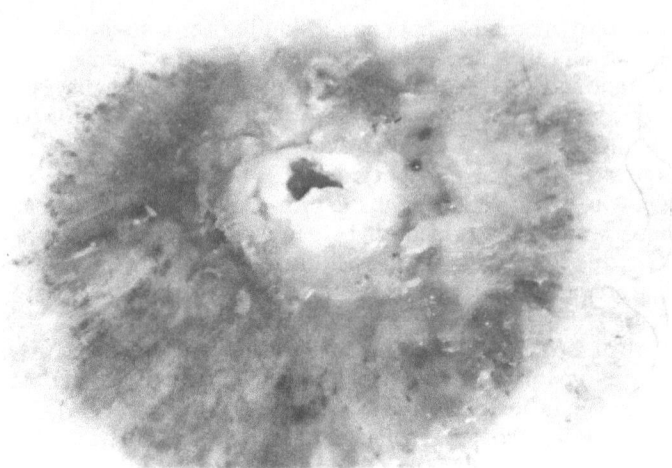

Fig.5.6. Flush ureterostomy—peristomal dermatitis caused by leakage.

Ulceration

Linear ulcers may be caused by pressure from a rigid plastic faceplate pushing against a long stoma which hangs over it into the collecting bag. Fear of damage to a longer stoma is often the cause of anxiety, and the curtailment of some sporting and social activities for many patients.

Peristomal Skin Irritation

Allergic reactions to adhesives, skin barriers and surgical tapes are a common cause of skin irritation, resulting in leakage and discomfort. Sensitive skin develops a characteristic area of erythema beneath the adhesive responsible, outlining the shape quite noticeably. Providing they themselves are not responsible, skin barriers such as Reliaseal, Karaya, Stomahesive and similar substances may be used to protect the skin. Folliculitis is a fairly common cause of skin irritation and infection beneath the faceplate of the urostomy appliance. It usually occurs in male patients who have hairy abdominal skin. These patients should be advised to shave or clip the hairs from the peristomal skin at regular intervals, taking care not to damage the stoma.

The gasket size of a urostomy appliance should not exceed the diameter of the stoma by more than 3 mm. If too large, the exposed peristomal skin, constantly bathed in urine, will develop the typical 'cobblestone' appearance of 'water-logged skin' (pseudo-epithelial hyperplasia) predisposing to infection, ulceration and eventual skin breakdown (Fig. 5.7). Too frequent removal of the urostomy appliance will also result in damage to the peristomal skin.

$\longrightarrow$

Fig.5.7. Pseudo-epithelial hyperplasia with typical 'cobblestone' appearance.

Fig.5.8. Phosphate deposits (ileal conduit).

Fig.5.9. Ileal conduit stoma following treatment for removal of phosphate deposits.

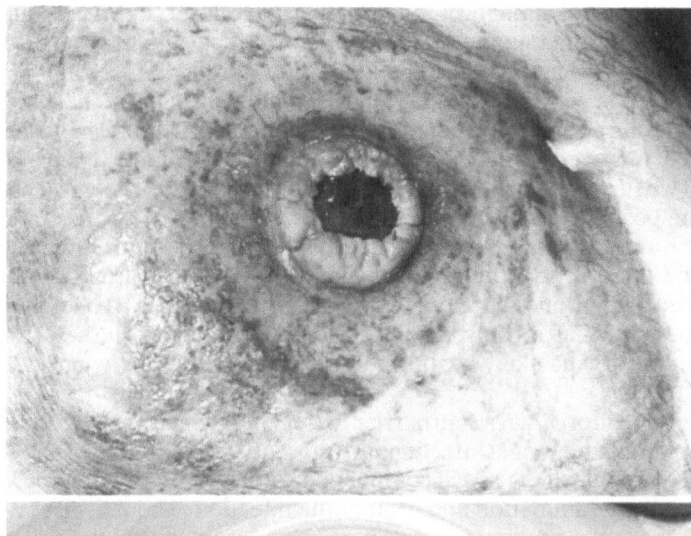

Fig.5.7.

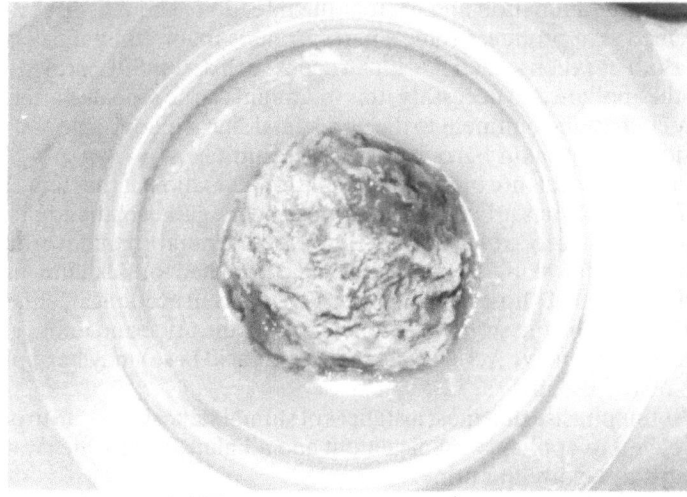

Fig.5.8.

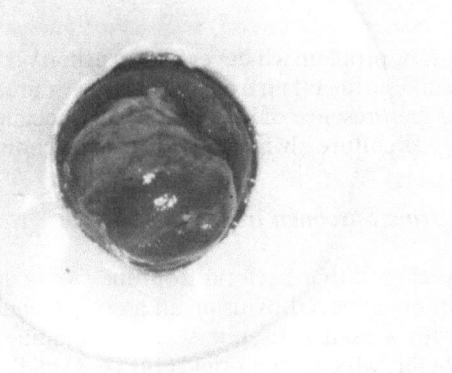

Fig.5.9.

Ideally, one-piece adhesive appliances, e.g. Coloplast, Hollister, Downs Rediflow, should be left in position for a minimum of three days and a maximum of seven days before changing, unless leakage occurs. The modern disposable 2-piece appliance, Surgical System 2, offers several advantages in that it combines a flange or base of skin barrier material, offering additional protection to the skin. The disposable pouches of this system can be removed and replaced without removal of the flange. It is particularly useful when access to the stoma is required to obtain a catheter specimen of urine and in the post-operative period.

The choice of urostomy appliance depends largely upon the individual requirements of each patient and there are various types available for use with urinary stomas; disposable, non-disposable, one-piece, or two-piece. The appliance of choice post-operatively must be one which is transparent, to allow observation of the new stoma, leakproof, non-irritant to the skin, comfortable to wear, and easily connected to overnight drainage.

Some patients require more than a skin barrier to treat peristomal skin excoriation, especially when bacterial and fungal infections are present. Triamcinolone (Adcortyl spray) is particularly useful when used in conjunction with nystatin powder or cream (Nystan) to reduce the inflammation and to treat the infection. The Adcortyl spray applied to the inflamed skin produces some smarting and is followed by the Nystan cream or powder. Both are then sealed in with an agent such as Op-Site spray which allows adhesion of the appliance. If necessary, this treatment can be repeated after 3–4 days. Applying oily creams and ointment to the peristomal skin is inadvisable as it will prevent the adhesion of most skin barriers, adhesives and tapes.

Deposits of phosphate crystals are often responsible for ulceration of the stoma and surrounding skin (Fig. 5.8). Friction between the stoma and the gasket of the appliance may occur and if ignored can lead to bleeding, infection and eventual breakdown of the mucosa and the peristomal skin. Poor hygiene and infected or alkaline urine predisposes to the formation of phosphate deposits. Five per cent acetic acid, either in the appliance or used to bathe the stoma will help to acidify the urine and remove the deposits (Fig. 5.9). Alternatively, Aci-jel Jelly (1% acetic acid base) may be applied to the stoma once or twice daily.

Bloom et al. (1981) emphasise that most instances of stomal stenosis are due to post-operative factors related to appliance management and alkaline urine. One gram of vitamin C daily helps to acidify the urine.

Urinary Infection

Urinary infection is a major problem whatever type of urinary diversion is selected. A sterile catheter specimen of urine taken from the conduit or ureterostomy for culture will confirm or exclude the presence of organisms. The specimen must not be taken from the collecting bag, as culture always yields a positive contaminated growth.

Method of Obtaining Urine Specimen from Ileal Conduit

Care must be taken to ensure that bacteria from the stoma are not introduced as contaminants. This can be achieved by using an aseptic technique and thoroughly cleansing the stoma with a mild antiseptic such as Betadine Solution. A female polythene residual catheter, which is semi-rigid (14FG or smaller) is inserted into the stoma, taking care not to be too forceful, as there is a small risk of perforating the ileum. A two-catheter technique is preferred (i.e. one catheter is introduced through the stoma and when in position, a second catheter is passed along the lumen to collect the specimen), but as yet this type of catheter is not available in Great Britain. If the catheter does not pass into the conduit easily, gentle pressure applied around the stoma will help the spout to protrude and admit the catheter.

The first few drops of urine should be discarded, and a sterile universal container used to catch the specimen.

Odour

Odour is not a major problem for urostomists, as it is for patients with colostomies or ileostomies. Most modern appliances are made from odourproof material which prevents the passage of odour through the bag. However, urine which develops a strong odour is often infected, and the patient should be encouraged to increase his fluid intake.

Various deodorising agents are available for use with ostomy appliances, but are of little value to the patient with a urinary stoma. Aerosol sprays such as Atmocol or Ozium are useful for freshening the air after each bag change.

Conclusion

It is hoped that the enthusiastic acceptance of stoma care nurses as an integral member of the surgical team, will prove of increasing value to our stoma patients and help restore their self-confidence in a return to an active and worthwhile life.

References

Bloom DA, Turner WR, Skinner DG (1981) Urological stomas. Modern technics in surgery. Urol Surg
Bricker EM (1950) Bladder substitution after pelvic evisceration. Surg Clin North Am 30: 1511–1521
Jeter KF (1976) Flush versus protruding urinary stoma. J Urol 116: 424–427
Jones MA, Breckman BB, Hendry WF (1980) Life with an ileal conduit: Results of questionnaire surveys of patients and urological surgeons. Br J Urol 52: 21–25
May HJ (1977) Enterostomal therapy. Raven Press, New York
Talbot JE (1975) Wakefield and District Postgraduate Medical Centre. A surgical diversion. Stoma care: A surgeons view p 45–50. Ed. by TK Clarke

Chapter 6

Urinary Reservoirs

Michael Handley Ashken

Introduction

If surgeons are to have a more radical approach to total cystectomy . . . it would be
clinically acceptable to surgeons and socially acceptable to patients if better methods of
urinary diversion could be offered. (Blandy 1964)

Is it worthwhile for our patients, to try and develop an appliance-free urinary
diversion, with a urinary reservoir, to be emptied by self-catheterisation? This is a
challenging question and justifies a small number of urologists throughout the world
studying a choice of viscus from which a urinary reservoir can be constructed, with
modifications in technique to try and make this type of diversion a viable alternative to
urinary conduits.

   This chapter aims to summarise the lines of thought taken by urologists during the
last thirty years in their quest to develop a continent urinary reservoir which is
technically acceptable to surgeons and socially acceptable to patients. A comparison
will be made of the advantages and disadvantages of using the ileocaecal segment, ileal
pouch or gastric pouch as the urinary reservoir. Emphasis will be given to pertinent
details of technique relating to the difficulties experienced in maintaining continence
and ease of catheterisation, with a variety of design valves constructed within the
reservoirs.

   Whilst an ileal conduit is currently the commonest and probably the least unsatisfactory proven urinary diversion performed throughout the Western World (Bricker
1957, 1980), there are many countries in the Middle East and Third World where a wet
cutaneous stoma is both socially and economically unacceptable. Bilharzia is
numerically the commonest known predisposing cause of bladder carcinoma, with
many patients throughout the world who could benefit if a reliable appliance-free
urinary diversion could be developed.

Ureterosigmoidostomy

The upper urinary tracts have been connected with virtually every conceivable viscus
(Hinman and Weyrauch 1936; Murphy 1972). The merit of any urinary reservoir must
be measured against a successful ureterosigmoidostomy. Every urologist will have a

small number of patients attending for follow-up with good results, having had a ureterosigmoidostomy by their predecessors 20–30 years earlier.

In this volume, Marberger and Straub have demonstrated the value of uretero-sigmoidostomy in children; and Walsh, the use of this technique in adults following radiotherapy in the preoperative treatment of malignant disease of the bladder. Goodwin and Scardino (1977) believed the operation of ureterosigmoidostomy was due for a renascence and Hanley, in his 1979 Bradshaw Lecture, advocated a reappraisal of ureterosigmoidostomy, because the earlier adverse criticisms (Irvine et al. 1956; Hopewell 1959) had followed a review of ureterosigmoidostomy being done by a number of surgeons using the Coffey technique (1911, 1931) without muco-mucosal anastomosis, or reflux prevention, in an era with few antibiotics and where metabolic absorption complications were poorly understood.

Jacobs (1967) had a large personal experience of ureterosigmoidostomy, using the improved mucosa to mucosa anastomosis, introduced by Nesbit (1949) and Cordonnier (1949). This, combined with submucosal tunnelling (Leadbetter 1951), produced results comparable to conduits and seems a reasonable technique to use in young adults or the elderly poor-risk patient, provided the overall renal function and upper renal tracts are normal, the ureters are not dilated, the large bowel is free of disease, the anal sphincter tone is good and there has not been a maximum radiotherapy dosage to the pelvis. It is acknowledged however that Riches (1967) found evidence of pyelonephritis or metabolic acidosis in 39.7% of 267 cases of ureterosigmoidostomy compared with 13% in 107 cases having ileal conduits. A 'three option' ureterosigmoidostomy as recommended by Turner-Warwick (1976) allows an easy conversion to a colostomy and rectal bladder or a colonic conduit if problems arise with pyelonephritis or metabolic acidosis. A palliative urterosigmoidostomy is useful, when the patient is likely to be dead from malignant disease before having time to become ill with pyelonephritis or metabolic acidosis, although many patients become incontinent and difficult to manage in the terminal stages.

There remains the anxiety of colonic neoplasia years after ureterosigmoidostomy (Whitaker et al. 1971; Trasti 1978). An increasing number of cases are being recorded in the literature following Hammers' (1929) original description. This risk raises a query about any urinary reservoir being constructed from large bowel in any patient having a good prognosis, although no case has been described of malignancy at a ureterocolic anastomosis where the faecal stream is not in contact with the anastomosis (Crissey et al. 1980) (see Chap. 4).

Continent Perineal Stoma

Any urinary reservoir with an abdominal wall stoma has the disadvantage of not having a true sphincter. To overcome this and also to avoid the well known complications of ureterosigmoidostomy, a number of technically ingenious operations have been reported, bringing faeces and urine through the anal sphincter to open on the perineum as separate ostia (Mauclaire 1895; Gersuny 1898; Heitz-Boyer and Hovelacque 1912; Lowsley and Johnson 1955; Stonington and Eiseman 1956; Rutishausger 1977; Tacciuoli et al. 1977; Ashken 1978b).

Gersuny's attempt in 1898 was greeted with scepticism which prevails today. Gersuny brought the mobilised pelvic colon behind the rectal bladder, to open on the perineum within the anal sphincter. Heitz-Boyer and Hovelacque (1912), pupils of Marion, modified Gersuny's operation bringing the pelvic colon anterior to the rectal bladder and their technique has gained popularity particularly in Italy as a urinary diversion in children with ectopia vesicae (Tacciuoli et al. 1977). Enthusiasm for this type of urinary diversion has not been maintained amongst American urologists and there is an ominous silence on any long-term follow-up in adult patients.

The author has a small experience (Ashken 1978b) using an ileocaecal urinary reservoir, drained by a separate length of ileum passing from the caecum to a perineal stoma anterior to the anal canal. This ileum was sleeved submucosally for about 10 cm within the anterior wall of the rectum and anal canal and within the levator ani and anal sphincters. This has the technical advantage over the Gersuny or Heitz-Boyer and Hovelacque operations in that if satisfactory perineal continence is not achieved, the ileocaecal reservoir can be easily isolated and rotated onto the anterior abdominal wall as a free draining conduit. The main technical problem is in mobilising the ileum on the superior mesenteric artery, to allow adequate length of the ileum to reach the perineum without tension.

In one of these cases, the mobilised ileum became ischaemic and sloughed; in a second case the patient had a fatal postoperative pulmonary embolus, whilst in a third case (Fig. 6.1), the perineal stoma remained healthy for 6 months until death occurred due to malignant disease. This patient was dry during the day, but had troublesome nocturnal incontinence as occurs in about 40% of patients with rectal bladders (Ghoneim and Ashamallah 1974). This problem of the wet or soiled bed makes any of these perineal stomas clinically suspect.

In general, this type of major reconstructive surgery is not favoured by most experienced urologists. It has no place with the neuropathic bladder; the loss of too much bowel from the alimentary tract may lead to malabsorption problems and in

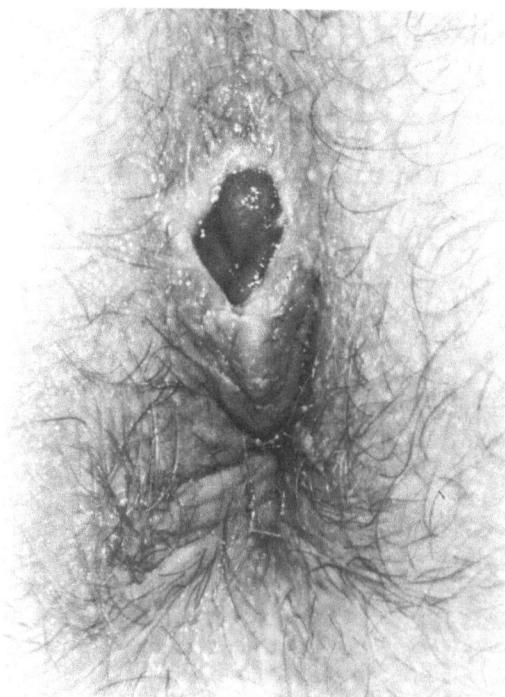

Fig. 6.1. Continent perineal ileostomy stoma anterior to anus. Does not retract as sometimes occurs with Gersuny type of perineal colostomy and rectal bladder.

malignant cases, extensive dissection is required within the irradiated pelvis. Even if this type of diversion is technically successful, Blandy (1961) has emphasised that 'hyperchloraemic acidosis must be a possible complication of a urinary reservoir constructed from any segment of bowel'.

Continent Abdominal Wall Stoma

The theoretical aims of any urinary reservoir are:

1) To be continent
2) To develop a good capacity at a low pressure
3) To be emptied easily by intermittent self-catheterisation
4) To preserve the upper renal tracts and maintain good renal function.
   The alimentary urinary reservoirs in current use with small numbers of patients are:
1) The caecum or ileocaecal segment (Gilchrist et al. 1950; Ashken 1974; Zingg and Tscholl 1977; Benchekroun 1977)
2) An ileal pouch (Norlen et al. 1974; Leisinger et al. 1975, 1976; Madigan 1976; Ashken 1980)
3) The stomach (Rudick et al. 1979).

Each viscus has its own advantages and disadvantages and these will be discussed in detail, although some of these procedures are of historical rather than practical importance, but illustrate the chain of thought in developing these diversions.

Techniques for Construction of Reservoir Valves, with Modifications to Prevent Eversion or Sliding of Valves

Ileocaecal Reservoirs

Gilchrist and his colleagues in Chicago (1950) have reported enthusiastically on their experience with the ileocaecal reservoir (Fig. 6.2). Continence depends upon the antiperistaltic function of the terminal ileum, the action of the ileocaecal valve and the small ileal skin stoma. Sullivan et al. (1973) reported their results in 40 patients with urinary reservoirs constructed between 1949 and 1963, with complete continence in 37 patients (94%). Unfortunately other workers have not had the same success.

Bricker (1950) and Bricker and Eiseman (1950) had experience with a similar ileocaecal urinary reservoir and found that true continence could not be achieved. Harper et al. (1954) using this technique in seven cases found their patients preferred to use an indwelling Foley catheter with intermittent evacuation of accumulated urine, whilst Brendler (1974 personal communication), after extending their New York series to 18 cases, confirmed that none of their patients were continent.

These misgivings about the continence of the natural ileocaecal valve or sphincter may explain why this type of urinary reservoir has not achieved common practical support amongst urologists, who have preferred the free-draining ileal conduit described at about the same time by Bricker (1950) in Missouri.

Gilchrist's original work has however acted as a catalyst to stimulate thought on the ileocaecal segment as a urinary reservoir, with modifications in technique to

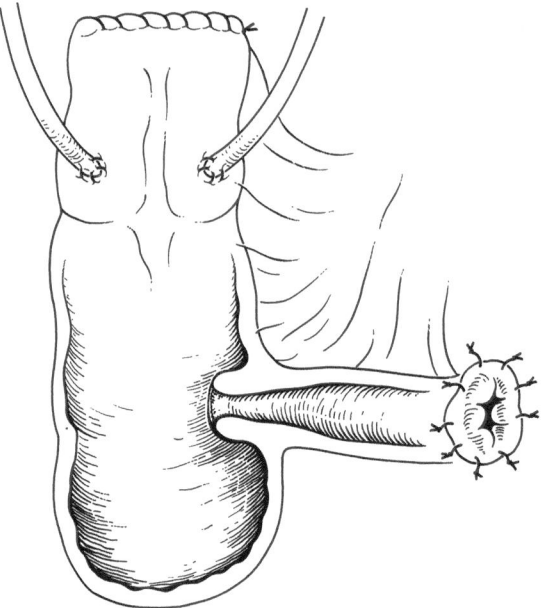

Fig.6.2. Caecal reservoir (Gilchrist). Continence of the ileocaecal valve is unreliable.

achieve an easily constructed and reliable valve within the reservoir. Having a personal preference for caecum in construction of a cystoplasty and experience of using the everted or spouted ileum as a reflux-preventing substitute for ureter when implanted into the bladder, a combination of these techniques was used (Ashken 1974) to construct a continent ileocaecal urinary reservoir.

Ileal Spout Valve

In the initial technique the ileocaecal segment was isolated, the ureters anastomosed into the terminal ileum using an intubated reflux-preventing split cuff and nipple technique (Turner-Warwick and Ashken 1967) and a separate *ileal spout valve* 5 cm in length was sutured into the open end of the caecum, to act as a competent valve (Fig. 6.3). The caecum around the ileal spout valve was anchored to the abdominal wall using four circumferentially placed non-absorbable sutures to buttress the reservoir, aiming to ensure a short and easy passage of a catheter into the reservoir via the skin flush ileostomy stoma (Fig 6.4).

Bowel continuity was restored with an end-to-end ileocolic anastomosis, the appendix removed and continuous drainage of the ureters and caecum maintained for 2 weeks. Intermittent catheterisation of the reservoir was then started initially 2-hourly, but extending within a few days to 4-hourly during the day and once at night (Fig. 6.5).

The general potential complications of all urinary reservoirs will be discussed later, but the specific and main complication of *eversion or sliding of the valve* will be discussed now.

Between 5 and 12 weeks postoperatively, four of the first seven cases developed prolapse of the ileal spout valve (Fig. 6.6), converting the continent reservoir into a free draining ileocaecal conduit. This was heralded by increasing difficulty with the self-catheterisation and some urinary incontinence.

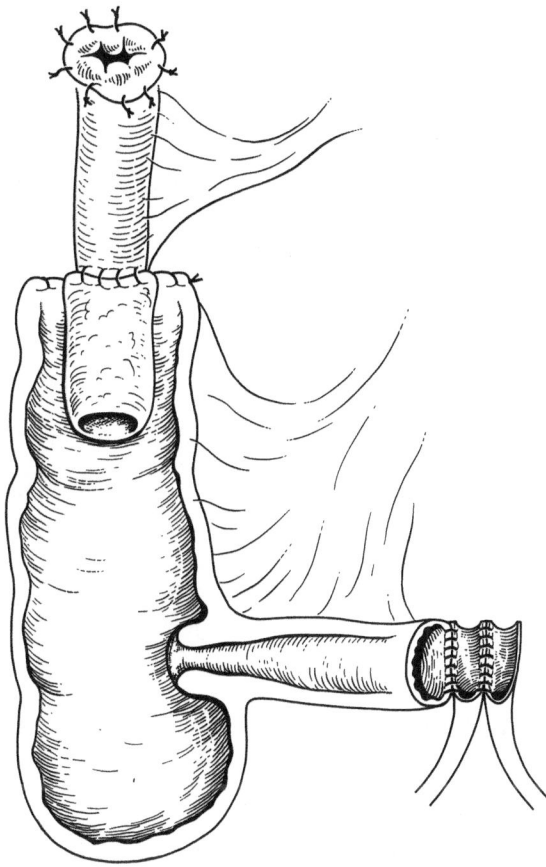

Fig.6.3. Ileocaecal reservoir with continent valve formed by everted spout of ileum (Ashken). Failed because of prolapse of the valve. Wallace ureteroileal anastomosis used in some cases.

What is the mechanism of this eversion prolapse and can it be prevented? On re-exploration in three cases, the ileal spouts looked healthy, without ischaemic or traumatic fibrosis but with very active peristalsis. The prolapse occurred in both isoperistaltic and retroperistaltic valves and was not prevented by a combination of superficial diathermy and suturing of the seroserosal surfaces and anchoring the ileal spout within the caecal reservoir. The latter sutures cut out with powerful peristaltic contraction of the spout valve as filling and distension of the reservoir occurred. Prolapse occurred for the second time within a few weeks in two of these cases after exploration and re-anchoring of the valve.

In a further four cases, the ileal spout valve was sutured within the caecum, having been sleeved through the true ileocaecal sphincter (Fig. 6.7). This anatomy had the disadvantage that the ureters were anastomosed directly into the caecum and were exposed to the high pressure waves within the reservoir and possibly partial ureteric obstruction by mucus collecting within the caecal sump. Two of these four cases still developed prolapse of the ileal spout about 8 weeks postoperatively. These spouts had to be excised to allow free drainage from the caecal conduit. One case did well on intermittent catheterisation for 8 months, but then presented as an emergency with a distended reservoir which could not be catheterised even under a general anaesthetic. The ileal spout was excised and revealed a significant submucosal haematoma from

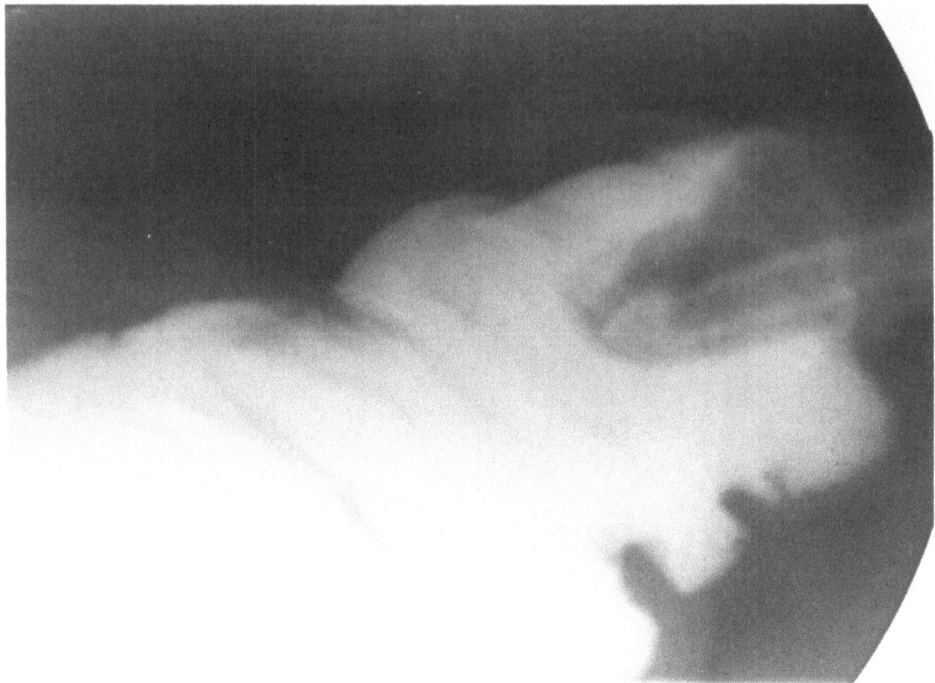

Fig.6.4. Caecogram showing competent ileal spout valve with empty catheter about to enter the caecal reservoir for drainage. Ashken 1974.

repetitive minor local trauma with the self-catheterisation. Due to increasing difficulty with the self-catheterisation, the fourth case elected to remain on continuous catheter drainage for over 2 years until his death from recurrent malignant disease. The catheter was changed every 2 weeks without urinary leakage.

Flutter Valve

The ileal spout valve was therefore simplified to a *'flutter valve'* with 5 cm of ileum hanging through the ileocaecal sphincter into the caecal reservoir (Fig. 6.8). In the two cases tried, both were continent. One died after 8 weeks with a myocardial infarction and the other died after 6 months with recurrent malignant disease, having used intermittent self-catheterisation during the day and continuous drainage at night. This helped improve his metabolic acidosis associated with impaired renal function.

The simplicity of the flutter valve was therefore combined with the original anatomical advantages of having the ureteroileal anastomoses protected by the true ileocaecal sphincter from the mucus and high pressure waves within the caecum. This reduced the risk of back pressure hydronephrosis, pyelonephritis and secondary metabolic acidosis. There is also no record of malignant change having arisen around any ureteroileal anastomosis. The ileal flutter valve may be sited through a taenia in the medial wall of the caecum or probably better, sewn into the open end of the caecum and this is the technique currently favoured by the author (Fig. 6.9), with 5 cm of the lateral wall of the caecum laid open and then closed with 2/0 Dexon, incorporating the antemesenteric border of the flutter valve to prevent sliding or prolapse of the valve.

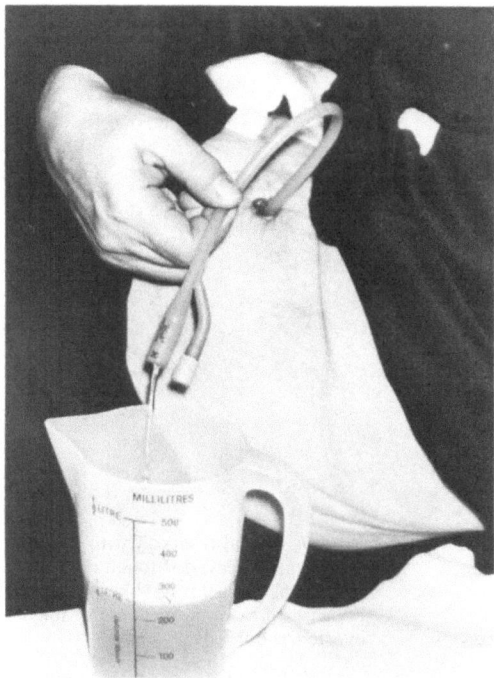

Fig.6.5. Self-catheterisation of a continent ileostomy stoma sited in the midline in preference to the right iliac fossa.

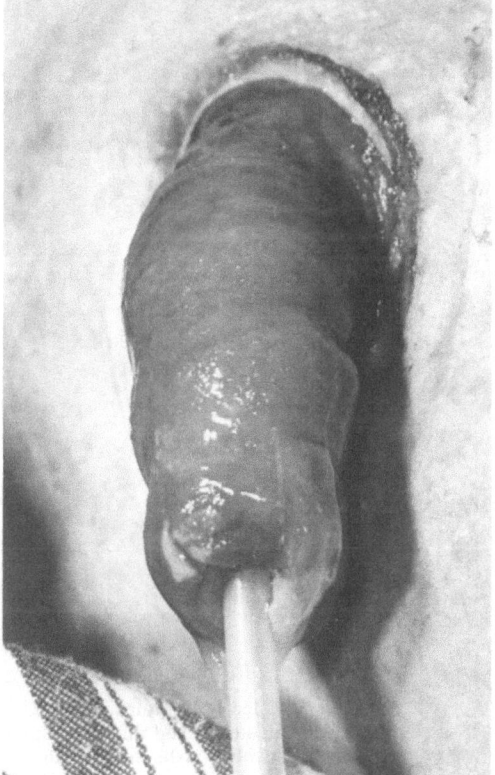

Fig.6.6. Prolapse of an everted spout valve from within an ileocaecal reservoir.

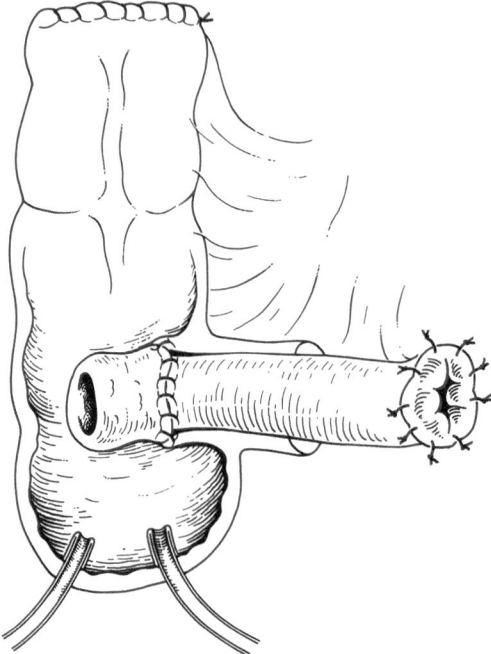

Fig.6.7. Caecal reservoir with everted spout valve sleeved through natural ileocaecal sphincter (Ashken). Also failed because of external prolapse of the everted spout valve.

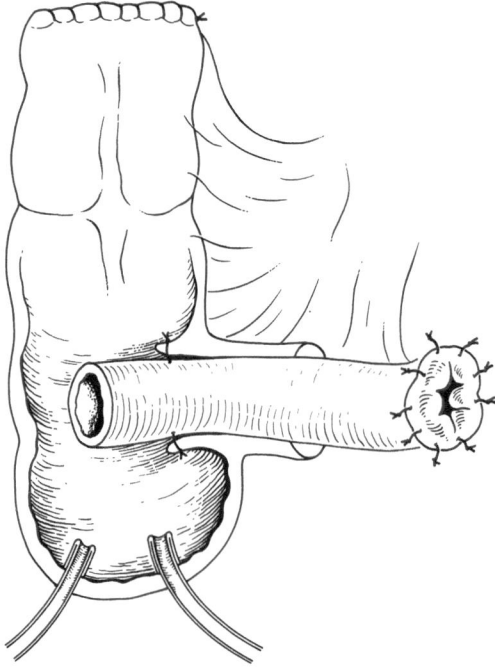

Fig.6.8. Caecal reservoir with flutter valve of ileum sleeved through natural ileocaecal valve (Ashken). Remains continent but with variable difficulty with catheterisation.

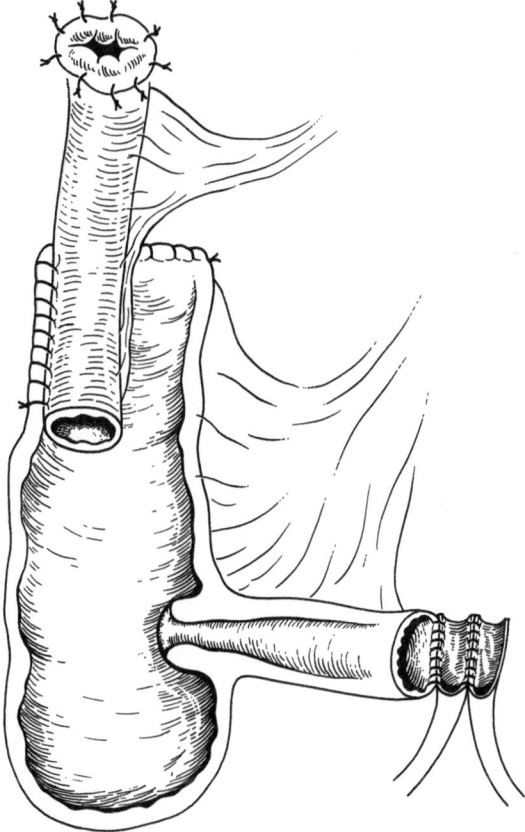

Fig.6.9. Ileocaecal reservoir with flutter valve sewn into open end of caecum (Ashken). Remains continent with easy intermittent self-catheterisation.

The remainder of the open end of the caecum is then closed with a continuous 2/0 Dexon suture to incorporate the valve and its mesentery. The skin flush ileostomy opening is deliberately made small to reduce the risk of later mucosal prolapse and minimise secretion on the surface.

The watertightness of the reservoir is tested by instilling saline into a catheter passed through the flutter valve. The initial capacity is about 150 ml, with a rapid increase to 400–500 ml within the first few postoperative weeks. Temporary drainage catheters are inserted as described in the original technique with daily washouts of 50–100 ml of a dilute bicarbonate solution to avoid mucus retention within the reservoir. The buttressing sutures between the caecum and inner aspect of the anterior abdominal wall must be placed carefully. In one case, the ileostomy was re-explored because a fibrous ridge had formed around a buttressing suture, making catheterisation difficult. This ridge was divided longitudinally and resutured transversely. At the same time, part of the subcutaneous ileum was plicated to avoid the catheter catching in an unsupported part of the ileal wall proximal to its entry into the caecum.

Following re-exploration, this case developed a small but persistent urinary fistula from the caecal reservoir close to the entry of the flutter valve. This valve was, therefore, excised, 3 months after its construction, converting the reservoir into a free-draining caecal conduit.

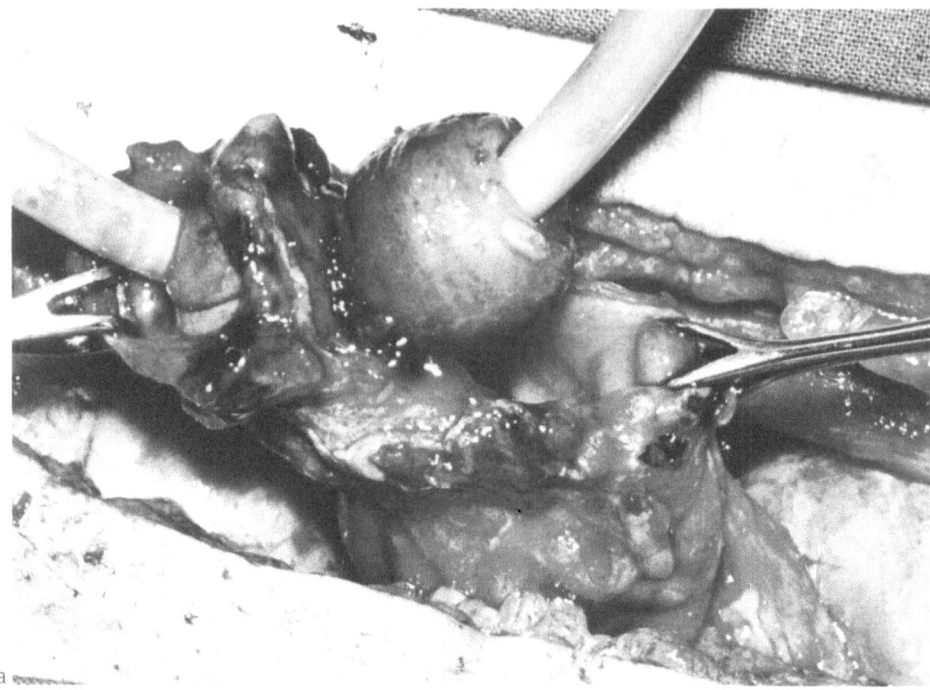

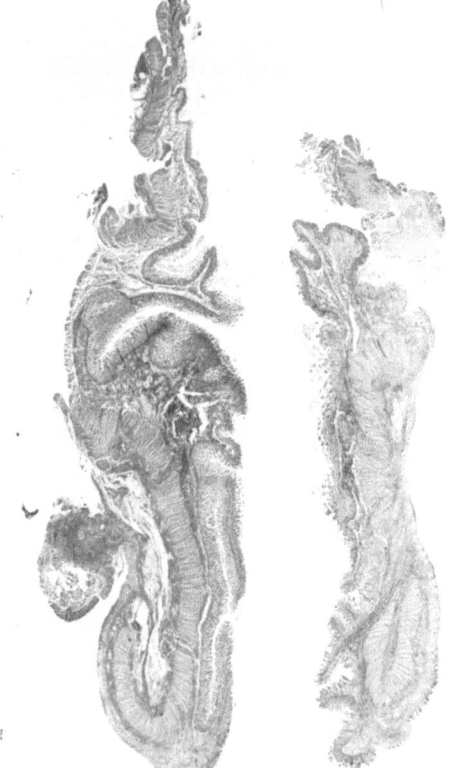

Fig.6.10. a Excision of flutter valve from caecal reservoir. The valve had become spout-shaped with a smooth surface and hung freely within the caecal reservoir. **b** Section of this flutter valve confirmed epithelialisation of the serosal surface and a surprising eversion of the free end of the valve including both mucosal and muscle layers.

Examination of the flutter valve was interesting. It had originally been 5 cm in length, with its antemesenteric border sewn into the lateral wall of the caecum. It was now conical or spout shaped, 2.5 cm in length and was no longer attached to the lateral wall of the caecum (Fig. 6.10a). The serosal surface was smooth with no sign of granulation tissue or inflammation. The wall of the valve had thickened, incorporating the mesentery to the valve in a smooth surface.

Splitting open the excised valve and histological studies revealed a surprising anatomy (Fig. 6.10b). The free open end of the flutter valve had everted itself at both mucosal and muscle layers. There was also some epithelialisation of the remaining external serosal surface with no sign of inflammation or ischaemia. These findings explained the naked eye thickening and shortening of the original valve and the smooth outer surface of the valve in constant contact with the urine in the reservoir.

With this spontaneous eversion of the tip of the flutter valve, subsequent prolapse onto the skin surface is considered much less likely than with the original deliberately everted spout valve. There were no signs of mucosal trauma or submucosal haemorrhage from the repetitive catheterisation of the valve.

Each patient will develop their own trick movements to achieve easy self-catheterisation, such as firm pressure and upward elevation of the abdominal wall immediately above the dry stoma, to counter the natural slight angulation where the flutter valve passes from the thickness of the anterior abdominal wall into the caecal reservoir.

The flutter valve has proven simple and reliable since first used in 1976 (Ashken 1978) and there has been only occasional intermittent problems with sliding of the valve. As, however, re-exploration has shown the flutter valve to shorten in length, its constructed length must be at least 5–7 cm to produce a permanent spout valve of over 2 cm which is the critical length to maintain continence. Although the valve does not remain sutured into the caecal wall, it is better to construct the flutter valve anchored within the reservoir to take up its natural position later and so avoid an early sliding of the valve. Use of colon for the flutter valve may avoid this sliding and eversion.

Ten of the initial 16 patients having an ileocaecal reservoir have died, mainly from recurrent malignant disease. Five of these patients had functioning reservoirs and five had been converted to free-draining caecal conduits because of spontaneous prolapse of the ilean spout valve or following surgical excision of the ileal valve because of increasing difficulty with self-catheterisation of the reservoirs.

Two female patients have managed well with flutter valves for over 5 years and one of these patients had already been converted from a urinary reservoir to a free draining caecal conduit. After 2 years she requested a re-conversion to a caecal reservoir, preferring intermittent catheterisation to the wearing of an ileostomy bag. They remain dry with healthy stomas and surrounding skin and with no deterioration in their upper renal tracts or renal function.

Intussusception Valve

Tscholl and Zingg (1977) in Berne have also had problems in trying to construct a competent valve within an ileocaecal reservoir. They used a technique similar to that described by Perl (1949), for a continent feeding jejunostomy, in which a *conical valve or nipple is made by intussusception of a bowel segment*. Smith and Hinman (1955) used this nipple for an 'intussuscepted ileal cystostomy' and found it to be continent.

Zingg and Tscholl (1977) used intussusception of the terminal ileum through the true ileocaecal sphincter, to hang as a nipple-shaped continent valve within the reservoir (Fig. 6.11). Whilst the initial results in four patients were encouraging, Zingg

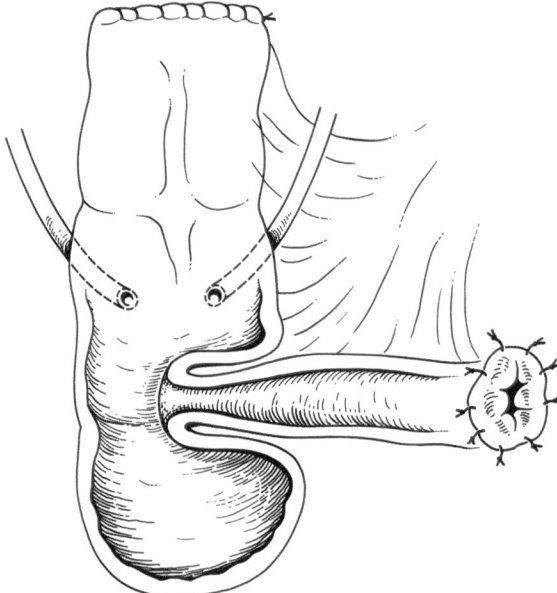

Fig.6.11. Caecal reservoirs with intussusception of terminal ileum through the natural ileocaecal sphincter (Zingg and Tscholl). Failed because of devagination of intussuscepted ileum.

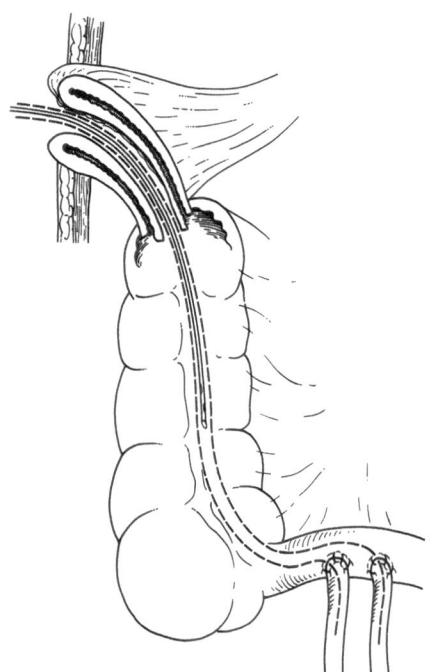

Fig.6.12. Ileocaecal reservoir with ink-well valve of ileum sewn into the open end of caecum (Benchekroun). Mesentery is exposed with risk of ischaemic necrosis of the valve.

(1978) reports that a sliding or devagination of the intussuscepted segment at the mesenteric border was a recurring problem. This is comparable to the experience of Kock and his colleagues, with sliding of the intussuscepted valves within an ileal pouch reservoir. Zingg concurs that a continent urinary reservoir can be constructed, but queries whether this will be to the benefit of our patients compared with a free draining conduit.

Ink-Well Valve

Encouraging results in the use of the ileocaecal urinary reservoir have been reported by Benchekroun (1977, 1980) working in Morocco. During 1974–1980, 32 patients had a caecal urinary reservoir and 29 (91%) were continent. Due to the hot climate and poor social conditions, a standard ileal conduit was unacceptable to these patients, particularly as the majority were young women following severe trauma to their lower urinary tracts secondary to prolonged and complicated labour of pregnancy.

In Benchekroun's series only three cases had bladder carcinoma. It is however significant, that almost half of the Moroccan patients had had a previous ileal conduit, ureterosigmoidostomy or rectal bladder with intractable complications justifying major reconstructive surgery to produce both a urologically and socially acceptable pattern of life.

Benchekroun uses an *'ink-well' design of ileal valve* sutured into the open end of the caecal reservoir (Fig. 6.12). As with other caecal reservoirs, prolapse of the 'ink-well valve' was the commonest complication, being reported in seven of 27 patients. Necrosis of the ileal valve required reconstruction in one case and in the author's only experience with the ink-well valve there was also some ischaemic necrosis of the valve with subsequent urinary leakage from the caecal reservoir. The skin surface ileostomy inevitably has a serosal covering with exposure of the fatty mesentery to the valve, risking local trauma and ischaemia.

Benchekroun recommends emptying the reservoir every 3–4 h because 12 patients had ureteric reflux with only 300–350 ml within the reservoir. This emphasises the unreliability of continence of the true ileocaecal sphincter when the pressure rises within the caecum due to distension with urine and superadded high pressure contraction waves of the caecum.

Benchekroun makes the interesting social observation that in Morocco, most patients cannot afford diversions with bags, whilst the wealthiest patients with urinary reservoirs only used each drainage catheter once.

Ileal Pouch Urinary Reservoirs

Whilst these modifications have been tried by a number of workers using ileocaecal reservoirs, Kock and his colleagues in Göteborg have extended their considerable pioneering experience with the continent ileal pouch in patients following total proctocolectomy, to a smaller number of patients having a continent ileal reservoir for urinary diversion using an intussusception valve (Kock et al. 1978b). The anatomy of this ileal pouch is very similar to that originally described by Blandy (1964) in his Hunterian Lecture on 'The feasibility of preparing an ileal substitute for the urinary bladder' (Fig. 6.13).

The Swedish workers have extensive experimental as well as clinical studies in the use of an ileal urinary reservoir. They set out to answer the following questions:

1) Whether the low-pressure volume capacity of the continent ileal reservoir would allow long enough intervals between catheterisation without back pressure obstruction to the upper renal tracts.

2) Would intermittent self catheterisation lead to urinary infection?

3) Would it be necessary to prevent ureteric reflux from the reservoir to the upper renal tracts?

4) Would metabolic disturbances occur from absorption through the ileal mucosa in the reservoir?

5) Would prolonged exposure to urine produce morphological changes in the ileal mucosa?

In their experimental work with dogs, Kock et al. (1978) showed that incontinence or reflux occurred if the intussuscepted valve was shorter than 11 mm whilst Leisinger et al. (1975) found reflux occurred if the valve was shorter than 19 mm. Intussuscepted valves were therefore constructed 20–30 mm in length, for on killing the dogs 12 weeks postoperatively, the upper renal tracts exposed to reflux were rapidly destroyed, whilst there were no severe pyelonephritic changes if reflux of infected urine was prevented.

Kock and his colleagues were encouraged with the answers to the other questions they had posed. They found that the ileal pouch rapidly developed a capacity of over 500 ml at pressures below 30 cm of water and that the urine usually remained sterile in spite of 4–6-hourly intermittent catheterisation. They demonstrated that prolonged contact of the ileal mucosa with urine produced an atrophy of the villi so that metabolic absorption problems did not occur and the surface area of the mucosa was greatly reduced. In most cases this is advantageous, but Nils Kock (1980, personal communication) reports that one of their patients never achieved a good capacity of her reservoir in spite of being continent. Blandy (1961) voiced this reservation about 'the possibility of delayed contracture and calcification of the pouch', following his extensive experimental surgery with an ileal pouch as a continent urinary reservoir, in which the mucosa and sub-mucosa had been removed to avoid metabolic absorption problems.

Just as both eversion of the ileal spout valve (Ashken 1974) or sliding of the intussuscepted ileal valve (Zingg 1978 personal communication) had been a serious technical problem in the ileocaecal reservoirs, so, sliding of the intussuscepted ileal valve tended to occur in the ileal reservoirs. Kock believed this was due to the bulk of mesentery between the two walls of the intussusception. This problem was originally highlighted by Smith and Hinman (1955) who implied that this sliding was cured by an adequate number of serosal sutures and roughening of the opposed serosal surfaces. There has been no evidence published to substantiate this hope.

Following their canine animal experiments Norlen et al. (1974) followed by Leisinger et al. (1976) and Madigan (1976) have constructed an ileal pouch reservoir in patients which has functioned physiologically with the encouraging results described in the earlier animal experiments.

In those patients converted from ileal conduits with skin and stoma problems, the 'quality of life' was much improved with a continent reservoir. The main complication however persisted, with a tendency for the intussuscepted valve to slide or devaginate making intermittent catheterisation difficult and the reservoir incontinent.

Kock et al. (1980) have done extensive animal experiments on new measures to maintain a stable intussuscepted valve and avoid devagination. After constructing a 5 cm long intussuscepted nipple valve, a GIA-staple gun loaded with special cartridges

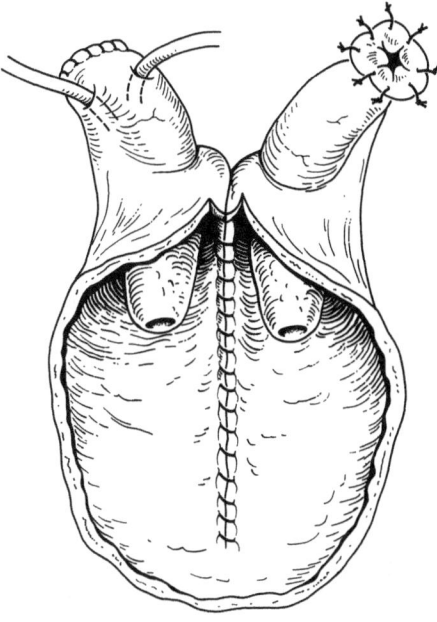

Fig.6.13. Ileal pouch reservoir (Kock). Difficulty in preventing devagination of intussuscepted nipple valves. This technique has been successfully extended, using the stapling gun on the valve and suturing strips of fascia or Marlex mesh around the base of the nipple.

is applied at four sites, two of them partly involving the mesentery. This is supplemented by suturing strips of fascia around the base of the nipple, or more recently, wrapping a 1.0–1.5 cm wide strip of Marlex mesh around the base of the nipple to prevent sliding of the valve.

Theoretically, the metal clips could slough into the reservoir and act as a nidus for stone formation. Histological studies, however, have shown that the staples were embedded in the muscular layer of the nipple and were completely covered by regenerated mucosa. At the site of the staples, the walls of the two intestinal segments forming the nipple were firmly fixed together by scar tissue.

Similarly, fibrous tissue had developed around the fascial strips or Marlex mesh to aid anchoring of the valve. Nipples constructed without staples, fascial strips or Marlex mesh showed little fibrous reaction. The space between the two segments remained filled with fat and loose connective tissue.

Cranley and McKelvey (1981) have done some interesting experimental studies in dogs and achieved a more reliable stable Kock intussuscepted valve. They combined techniques of mesenteric exclusion and marginal artery preservation with deep seromuscular diathermy to produce a good circumferential fibrous union between the layers. They found construction of the valve with the autosuture GIA stapling gun shortened the operating time but did not improve valvular stability. Cranley and McKelvey emphasise that their technique of mesenteric exclusion has only been used in isolated bowel and has not been used in clinical practice where there is a theoretical risk of endangering the blood supply of this valve when constructed within a bowel reservoir.

Since 1975 Nils Kock (1980, personal communication) has used an ileal pouch as a continent urinary diversion in 11 patients. One patient died in an accident and the remaining ten patients are continent and their ileal reservoirs are functioning well.

Kock believes 'that this method for urinary diversion will have its place in surgery as an alternative to other procedures', and is optimistic that improved surgical technique to avoid devagination of the valve will reduce the incidence of complications to an acceptable level. However, the extent of the reconstructive surgery needed to construct any continent urinary reservoir is likely to detract from its widespread use as a method for urinary diversion, particularly if combined with a total cystectomy. Nils Kock (1980, personal communication) agrees that the caecal reservoir is more easily constructed, but feels that the pressure developed within the caecal reservoir could, in the long term, have an adverse effect on the upper renal tracts.

As an alternative to try to overcome this real technical problem with either the everted spout or intussuscepted valves, the author has combined the metabolic and volume pressure advantages of the Kock ileal pouch with the use of the simple *flutter valve* already proven to maintain continence, with little risk of prolapse or sliding when used with the caecal reservoir (Ashken 1978).

An ileal pouch reservoir is constructed as described by Kock et al. (1978) and as used by Leisinger et al. (1976) and Madigan (1978) using about 40 cm of ileum selected about 25–30 cm from the ileocaecal valve to avoid later malabsorption and vitamin B_{12} deficiencies.

Instead of intussuscepting ileum into the two limbs of the pouch to act as valves, a 10-cm length of ileum isolated on its blood supply is sleeved into the pouch to produce a 5-cm flutter valve within the reservoir. The proximal end of this flutter valve will later form the continent skin flush ileostomy.

Both animal experimental and clinical work has shown that it is safer to anastomose the flutter valve directly and freely into the pouch. If the flutter valve is pulled through a limb of ileum entering or leaving the pouch, its blood supply may be impaired.

Donnelly (1981) working in Dublin, has done some interesting studies in dogs with continent ileal pouch urinary reservoirs. In an initial series of six dogs, Donnelly reports that four were continent up to volumes of 400 ml of urine. He found the flutter valve simple to construct and that the free end of the flutter valve hanging within the reservoir turns itself back with eversion for about 1 cm to shorten the functional length of the valve exactly as noted by Ashken (Fig. 6.9a,b) with a caecal reservoir.

Two of the seven dogs died with gangrene of the flutter valve. Others had a fibrous ring where the valve was sleeved through the ileum into the pouch leading to distension and then a kinking obstruction of the ileum outside the pouch with a back-pressure hydronephrosis and renal failure. Donnelly therefore recommends other methods to avoid reflux and obstruction such as a submucosal or seromuscular tunnelling of the ureters. This saves having to construct a second flutter valve for anastomosis of its proximal end to the ureters.

When a standard ileal conduit is converted to a continent reservoir the original ureteroileal anastomoses can be left intact. The distal end of the conduit is sleeved into the newly constructed ileal pouch as the second flutter valve.

Should there be a technical failure of the skin surface flutter valve, it can be excised and a further segment of ileum isolated on its blood supply and sewn as a flutter valve into the otherwise satisfactory ileal reservoir. Alternatively, an ileal pouch reservoir can be easily managed with an indwelling Foley balloon catheter on continuous drainage. This is being used by the author in one adult case with a closed meningo-myelocele, severe kyphoscoliosis and repeated failed readjustments of a free-draining ileal conduit stoma, where a satisfactory urostomy bag could not be fitted (Fig. 6.14a,b). Whilst on intermittent catheterisation, overfilling of the ileal pouch reservoir had been an intermittent problem because of a diminishing sensation of distension within the reservoir. He uses either 3-hourly intermittent or continuous catheter drainage as he wishes (Fig. 6.14c,d).

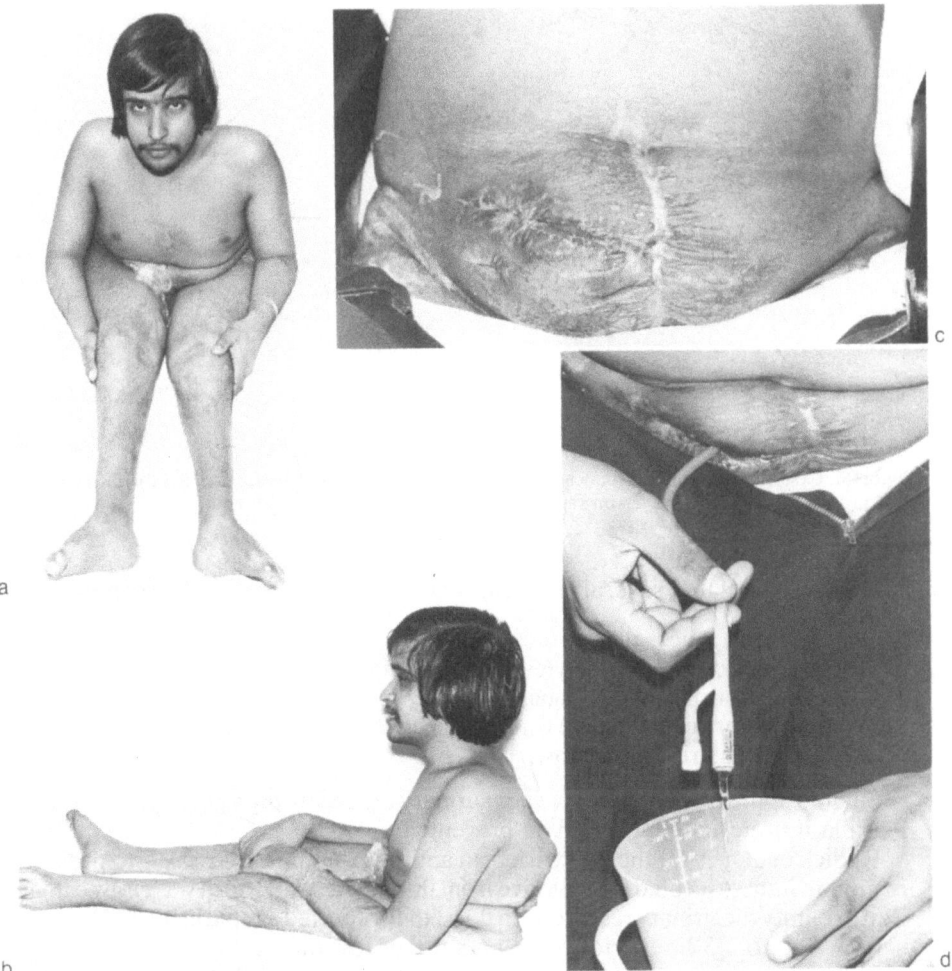

Fig.6.14. a, b Ileal conduit stoma problems in a patient with severe kyphoscoliosis. **c** Dry ileostomy stoma after conversion to a continent ileal pouch reservoir with flutter valves. **d** Self-catheterisation of flutter valve in ileal pouch reservoir.

Gastric Reservoirs

The principle of an intussusception valve as used by Kock in the ileal pouch has been reproduced by Rudick et al. (1977) using the vagally denervated gastric fundus as a urinary reservoir.

Sinaiko (1960) constructed an artificial bladder using a gastric pouch in both dogs and humans, to try and avoid the long-term potential metabolic absorption problems where urine is in contact with colonic mucosa and to a lesser extent with ileal mucosa (Schmidt et al. 1973).

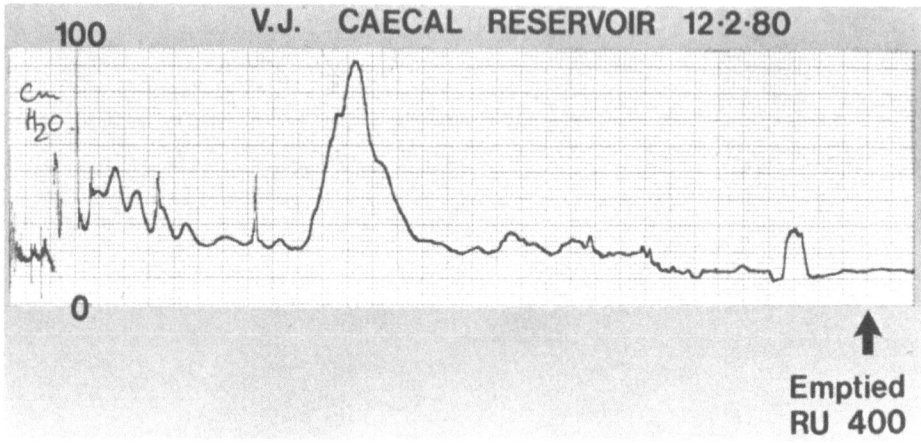

Fig.6.15. Cystometrogram with ileocaecal reservoir. Low basal and filling pressures with superadded high pressure contraction waves on rapid filling of reservoir.

Sinaiko postulated several theoretical advantages of using a gastric pouch:

1) The stomach mucosa is practically non-absorbing.
2) There is no loss of electrolytes, such as potassium.
3) Gastric secretions protect against urinary infection.
4) No ureteric or renal damage was noted and the proximal ureter could be used for the ureterogastric anastomosis.

Sinaiko appreciated that a continent urinary bladder using a gastric pouch was only feasible if ureteric reflux could be prevented.

Rudick et al. (1977) therefore used an antireflux ureterogastric anastomosis and a continent intussuscepted nipple valve from the gastric wall, which was easily catheterised to empty the urinary reservoir. In dogs, they reported a rapid increase in reservoir capacity up to 1.5 litres with a low pressure of less than 12 cm H_2O.

Following their canine experiments, Rudick et al. (1979) have a small clinical experience, with the human gastric pouch again developing a good capacity at a low pressure. Serum electrolytes remained normal and the histological secretory and permeability characteristics of the pouch remained unchanged with prolonged exposure to urine. The urine remained sterile, for the acid content and gastric lysozyme inhibit bacterial growth. The pouch can be sited in the upper abdomen away from any pelvic irradiation and a short length of proximal ureter can be used for the ureterogastric anastomosis.

The main challenge to the success of any urinary reservoir operation remains maintaining continence and easy self-catheterisation.

Intussusception Valve

Any *intussusception nipple valve*, whether into a caecal, ileal or gastric reservoir, will tend to slide and devaginate. The number and ingenuity of techniques described to try and avoid this complication confirms the seriousness of the problem. Whilst Leisinger et al. (1975) state that 'the construction of intussuscepted nipple valves is easy', Kock et al. (1978) stress that 'the construction of valves which remain competent is far from easy'. The same criticism applies to the *everted ileal spout valve*.

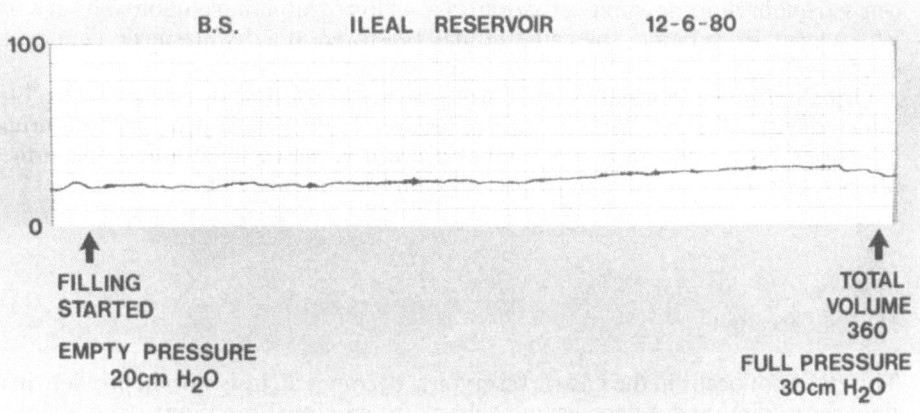

Fig.6.16. Cystometrogram with ileal pouch reservoir showing very low pressure with filling to 360 ml.

Peristalsis remains very active within these ileal valves and combined with episodes of bowel spasm precipitated by the repetitive minor local trauma of the self-catheterisation, contributes to the valves' eversion or slide. This complication occurs in valves constructed in both an isoperistaltic or retroperistaltic direction.

Another adverse factor to the continence and anatomy of these valves is the pressure waves within the urinary reservoir, particularly in the caecal cases. Occasional intermittent caecal contractions may reach an unsubtracted pressure of 80–100 cm H_2O but there is only a slowly rising pressure within the caecal reservoir as distension occurs, and superadded contraction waves are rare when filling is slow (Fig. 6.15). The pressure patterns within the ileal and gastric reservoirs are even more favourable, with only a slow and relatively small rise in unsubtracted pressure from 10–30 cm H_2O, in spite of achieving capacities of over 500 ml (Fig. 6.16).

Potential Complications of Urinary Reservoirs

In any urinary reservoir drained by intermittent catheterisation, potential complications include urinary infection, mucus secretion, stone formation and metabolic absorption abnormalities. In practice, these complications vary with the type of reservoir constructed and these differences will be compared and contrasted.

Urinary Infection

In the self-catheterisation of urinary reservoirs, a socially clean but not always bacteriologically sterile catheter is used, comparable to the currently favoured intermittent catheterisation of the neuropathic bladder (Lapides et al. 1974, 1976). The catheter most commonly used is an 18–20F folatex catheter or Nelaton catheter. Some patients find the latter too stiff, with the risk of perforation or pain on introducing the catheter. A single catheter may be used for 1–2 weeks and after use is washed under running water and stored in cetavlon or hibitane solution when at home. When away from home, the catheter may be stored in a dry plastic or Tupperware container.

Urine cultures are usually sterile from the gastric or ileal reservoirs, whilst often infected with coliforms from the caecal reservoirs. Proteus or pyo-cyaneous urinary infections have been rare. Antibiotics are not recommended unless the urine is offensive or there are systemic signs and symptoms of infection.

Mucus Secretion

This does not occur in the gastric reservoirs, becomes an insignificant problem in the ileal reservoirs, and a decreasing problem in the caecal reservoirs. In the author's cases, serial biopsies of the reservoir walls show no change in the columnar epithelium lining the caecal reservoirs in spite of several years of continuous contact with urine and there is a persistence of mucus-secreting cells in the caecum. This is in contrast to changes in the caecal wall noted by Brendler (1974 personal communication) who biopsied the caecum in one case after about a year and found the epithelium had undergone metaplasia to the transitional type. Attempts to reduce mucus secretion by the local introduction of Yttrium 80 into the large bowel failed and Irvine et al. (1960) actually reported an increase in mucus secretion due to irritation from the hypertonic β-ray emitting material.

The ileal mucosa behaves very differently with prolonged contact with urine. Atrophy of the villi occurs within a few months, reducing both its secretory and absorptive area.

Mucus secretion within the caecal reservoirs may contribute to hypokalaemia and mucus retention to urinary infection. Weekly reservoir washouts with sterile water or bicarbonate solution are recommended to avoid mucus retention. Temporary blockage of the catheter during drainage of the reservoir is usually easily cleared by the patient coughing or straining to momentarily raise the intra-abdominal and intra-reservoir pressure. The persistence of mucus secretion makes it more difficult to manage caecal reservoirs with selective continuous drainage as an alternative to intermittent catheterisation. Blockage of the drainage catheter risks overdistension of the reservoir, but spontaneous perforation has not occurred. Fortunately, patients retain the sensation of distension within the caecum as filling occurs, whilst sensation is sometimes diminished within the ileal pouch reservoir.

Stone Formation

Urinary stasis, residual urine and mucus retention in a bowel reservoir can predispose to stone formation within the reservoir. Benchekroun (1980) reported stones within caecal reservoirs in six of 27 cases and Leisinger (1979) noted large stones in a patient after 2 years with an ileal pouch reservoir. The stone was removed by open operation. No stones have been recorded in the upper renal tracts or ureters amongst patients with reservoir diversions. Litholapaxy for small stones within a reservoir should be possible under direct vision, with care not to perforate the relatively thin viscus wall. No reservoir stones have developed so far in my own cases.

Metabolic Abnormalities

Hyperchloraemic acidosis and lowering of the whole body potassium (Williams et al. 1967) were common complications with long-standing ureterosigmoidostomy (Jacobs and Barr Stirling 1952). This was partly due to the early cases having a Coffey ureterocolic anastomosis which allowed reflux pyelonephritis and ureteric stenosis in a pre-antibiotic era. Grey Turner (1929) had shown that with ureterosigmoidostomy urine collected right round to the caecum, exposing a vast area of colonic mucosa to urine through which urea and chloride were absorbed.

As with ureterosigmoidostomy, the success of any appliance-free urinary diversion depends on having normal upper renal tracts which can compensate for absorption of metabolites across mucous membranes and retain normal renal function and serum electrolytes (see Chaps. 3 and 4).

Whilst Sullivan et al. (1973) have not reported any significant hyperchloraemic acidosis in their caecal reservoirs, the author has found a laboratory shift to a slightly raised serum chloride and lowered serum bicarbonate after 3–4 years with a continent ileocaecal reservoir. This can be countered successfully by oral sodium bicarbonate 2 G q.i.d. with meals and if necessary by more frequent catheterisation of the reservoir during the day and continuous drainage at night. If metabolic acidosis does occur, an intravenous urogram must be done to check the drainage of the upper renal tracts.

Metabolic acidosis and loss of potassium do not occur in the ileal and gastric reservoirs. In the former, Hansson et al. (1978) have done extensive morphological studies using both light and electron microscopy to record the changes in the ileal mucosa lining the reservoirs. After 1 year, there was a loss of villous elements with regressive changes reducing the absorptive area. Although the urine was usually sterile it was toxic to the ileal mucosa. This is in contrast to the caecal mucosa with prolonged contact with urine where the columnar epithelium and mucus glands persist. Rudick et al. (1979) found that with gastric urinary reservoirs, urine produced no change in the histological, secretory or permeability characteristics of the gastric mucosa and hence no metabolic absorption disturbance.

Urinary Fistula

If an early postoperative urinary fistula develops around the valve in an ileocaecal reservoir, it is likely that the valve will eventually have to be excised and either reconstructed or the reservoir converted into a free draining caecal conduit. Continuous catheterisation usually fails to heal this fistula because of both frequent blockage by mucus and intermittent high pressure caecal contractions forcing urine through the fistula and sometimes expressing the catheter from the reservoir.

Conversely, a urinary fistula from an ileal pouch reservoir usually heals with continuous catheter drainage. There is less mucus to cause blockage of the catheter and the pressures within the ileal pouch are lower than within the caecum. The intussuscepted Kock valve avoids a vulnerable suture line as is constructed with a caecal reservoir and is a technical factor favouring the ileal pouch reservoir.

The caecal reservoirs have the attraction of being ready made and technically simpler, and may therefore be preferable when combined as a one-stage urinary diversion with total cystourethrectomy or anterior pelvic exenteration, particularly where there are contraindications to a ureterosigmoidostomy. In the long term, the theoretical disadvantages of the caecal reservoirs are the persistence of mucus secretion, urinary tract infections and the occasional high intraluminal pressures associated with intermittent contraction waves within the caecal wall.

In spite of the theoretical advantages of using the denervated gastric fundus as a reservoir, most urologists are likely to remain reluctant to interfere with a normal stomach as part of an already major operation, for fear of potential post-operative gastric complications. Even Rudick et al. (1979) have reported fistulae, bowel obstruction and ureteric obstruction in their small series. I therefore feel that it is unlikely that many surgeons will wish to include this complicated technique in their repertoire of urinary diversions.

Conclusion

In the author's opinion 'it is worthwhile for our patients, to try and develop an appliance-free urinary diversion with a urinary reservoir, to be emptied by self-catheterisation'. The present indications however still remain limited and further long-term follow-up of a number of patients remains essential before this type of urinary diversion can be recommended for general use as a viable and sensible alternative to more established techniques.

A urinary reservoir and appliance-free urinary diversion should be considered in the following circumstances:

1) In patients with a urinary conduit where there are intractable stoma complications making it impossible to fit a urostomy bag to keep the patient dry and the surrounding skin healthy in spite of the skills of a stomatherapist. This may apply particularly to patients with a neuropathic bladder where their shape and posture make it impossible to site and fit a urostomy appliance. Some patients having multiple sclerosis with involvement of their hands, making changing of their urostomy bags difficult, might find it easier to do self-catheterisation of a urinary reservoir.

2) In patients who for social, emotional or economic reasons would or do find a wet stoma unmanageable or unacceptable.

3) Some cases requiring palliative urinary diversion due to intolerable lower tract urinary symptoms in which the upper renal tracts are normal but in whom the bladder is inoperable or does not need removal.

4) As an elective urinary diversion in women with severe urinary incontinence in whom less drastic measures have failed. Similarly, in the rarer incontinent male patient where problems with the penis, urethra or bladder exclude management of the incontinence with a catheter, penile appliance, prosthesis or clamp.

A urinary reservoir is contraindicated in very obese patients due to both technical problems experienced with the bowel mesentery in construction of the reservoir or its competent valve and later difficulty with introducing the drainage catheter into the reservoir through the thick anterior abdominal wall. It is also unwise to construct a urinary reservoir if there is already significant impairment of renal function and a creatinine clearance of less than 50 ml/min.

The main practical choice is between using the ileocaecal segment or an ileal pouch reservoir. It will be valuable for all of us, if a small number of different Urological Units persevere with their different techniques until the indications, successes and failures are clarified. The results of both Benchekroun in Morocco and Kock in Sweden are particularly encouraging, but no one technique for a continent urinary reservoir is clearly better than the others. There are advantages and disadvantages in using either the ready made ileocaecal segment or the surgically constructed ileal pouch.

My present personal preference is to use the ileocaecal reservoir with a competent flutter valve for the following reasons:

1) The ileocaecal segment is ready made and the right shape.

2) The ureteroileal anastomosis lies outside the main caecal reservoir and is to some extent protected from any infection or pressure within the caecal reservoir by the natural ileocaecal valve or sphincter.

3) The flutter valve is much simpler to construct than an ink well valve or any intussusception valve and minimises the serious complication of sliding or de-vagination of the valve. Its constructed length must allow for some contraction of the valve.

4) The flutter valve is made from a short segment of ileum on a good blood supply contiguous to where the terminal ileum is divided for the ureteroileal anastomosis. Tailored colon may prove better for construction of the flutter valve.

5) The ileocaecal segment and ileum used for the flutter valve is unlikely to have been damaged by any preoperative irradiation to the pelvis.

6) Whilst coliforms can frequently be cultured from the reservoir urine, clinical pyelonephritis is rare.

7) Although mucus secretion persists, it tends to slowly diminish and if weekly washouts of the reservoir are done mucus retention and stone formation should not be a problem.

8) A good capacity reservoir develops rapidly and sensation within the caecum avoids over-distension.

9) Any tendency to hyperchloraemic acidosis can be countered with oral bicarbonate or potassium citrate.

10) The anatomy of the ileocaecal segment allows a simple conversion to a free-draining caecal conduit if necessary.

In contrast, the ileal pouch requires considerably more reconstructive surgery which detracts from the technique if combined with a total cystourethrectomy. If pre-operative radiotherapy has been given, the small bowel selected for the pouch may be compromised by irradiation changes which may not be obvious to the operator. There are more suture lines to heal and a greater length of ileum is removed from the alimentary tract. There are, however, definite physiological advantages of the ileal pouch over the ileocaecal segment. Atrophy of the ileal mucosal villi reduces the secretion of mucus, the risk of absorptive metabolic acidosis and probably explains why the urine is often sterile within an ileal pouch. This pouch develops a good capacity with low intraluminal pressures, but the sensation of distension is not always as reliable as with the caecal reservoir.

Because the construction of any urinary reservoir takes longer than a standard conduit and does have an increased morbidity and technical complications, it is unlikely that it will ever replace a urinary conduit as the first choice for urinary diversion in most cases, particularly when combined with major ablative surgery for malignant disease where preoperative full dosage radiotherapy has been given. I am however optimistic that the ileocaecal segment and a flutter valve are simple enough to construct to make this a viable practical operation (Fig. 6.17a,b).

It will take at least a 10-year follow-up to reveal whether or not any appliance-free urinary diversion will concur with Bricker's (1950) dictum 'that urinary continence must not be achieved to the detriment of renal function'. The final verdict will rest with our patients, to say and demonstrate whether or not these procedures are a worthwhile

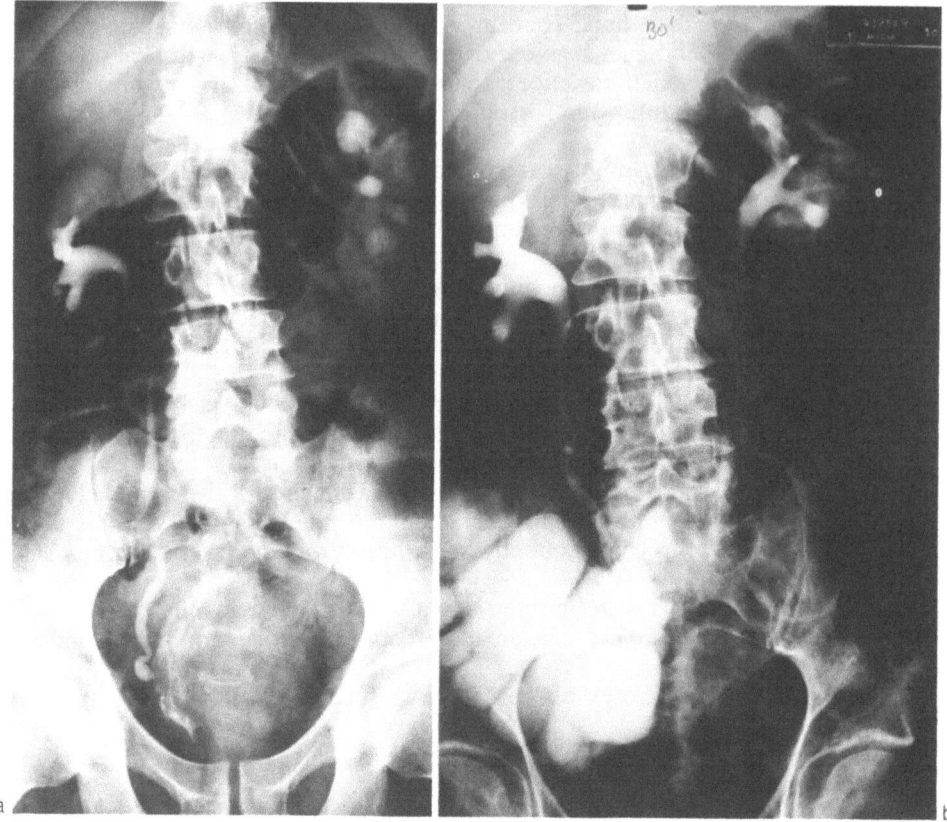

Fig. 6.17. a Intravenous urogram with a large bladder carcinoma obstructing the left ureter. **b** Intravenous urogram three months after cystectomy with resolution of the left hydronephrosis and filling of the continent ileocaecal reservoir. Ashken 1974.

advance or a complicated failure, to be discarded to the historical archives of condemned surgical technique (Fig. 6.18).

Urologists should at least be able to contemplate construction of a urinary reservoir type of diversion in selected patients, for one of the themes of this volume is to encourage the surgeon to select the type of urinary diversion most appropriate to any individual patient, echoing the clinical approach of Blandy (1970) in his comprehensive review on urinary diversion. We will wish to avoid the situation so poignantly put by Hanley in his Bradshaw Lecture, that 'following some urinary diversions, life is prolonged plus misery'. This must act as a stimulus and justify at least a small number of urologists throughout the world to strive to improve on the least unsatisfactory techniques available to us today.

References

Ashken MH (1974) An appliance-free ileocaecal urinary diversion: Preliminary communication. Br J Urol 46: 631–637
Ashken MH (1978a) Continent ileocaecal urinary reservoir. J R Soc Med 71: 357–360

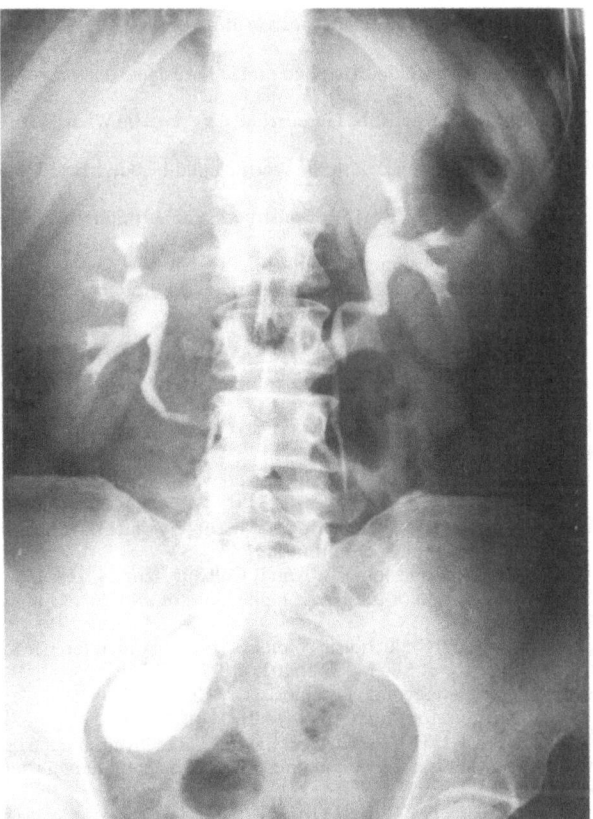

Fig.6.18. Intravenous urogram 5 years after diversion into an ileocaecal reservoir with a continent flutter valve and normal renal function.

Ashken MH (1978b) The continent urostomy. Br Med J ii: 830

Benchekroun A (1977) Continent caecal bladder. Eur Urol 3: 248–250

Benchekroun A (1980) Continent caecal bladder. Br J Urol (awaiting publication)

Blandy JP (1961) Ileal pouch with transitional epithelium and anal sphincter as a continent urinary reservoir. J Urol 86: 749–767

Blandy JP (1964) The feasibility of preparing an ileal substitute for the urinary bladder. Ann R Coll Surg Eng 35: 287–311

Blandy JP (1970) Methods of urinary diversion and replacement of the bladder. In: Riches Sir E (ed) Modern trends in Urology. Butterworths, London, pp 180–203

Bricker EM (1950) Bladder substitution after pelvic evisceration. Surg Clin North Am 30: 1511–1521

Bricker EM (1957) The technic of ileal segment bladder substitution. Progress in Gynaecology 3: 695–712

Bricker EM (1980) Current status of urinary diversion. Cancer 45: 2986–2991

Bricker EM, Eiseman B (1950) Bladder reconstruction from cecum and ascending colon following resection of pelvic viscera. Ann Surg 132: 77–84

Coffey RC (1911) Physiologic implantation of the severed ureter or common bile-duct into the intestine. JAMA 56: 397–403

Coffey RC (1931) Transplantation of the ureters into the large intestine. Submucous implantation method. Personal studies and experiences. Br J Urol 3: 353–428

Cordonnier JJ (1949) Ureterosigmoid anastomosis. Surg Gynecol Obstet 88: 441–446

Cranley B, McKelvey STD (1981) The Kock ileostomy reservoir: an experimental study of methods of improving valve stability and competence. Br J Surg 68: 545–550

Crissey MM, Steele GD, Gittes RF (1980) Rat model for carcinogenesis in ureterosigmoidostomy. Science 207: 1079–1080

Ferris DO, Odel HM (1950) Electrolyte pattern of the blood after bilateral ureterosigmoidostomy. JAMA 142: 634–640

Gursuny R (1898) Cited by Foges: Officielles protokll der K.K. Gesellschaft der Aertze in Wien. Wien Klin Wochenschr 11: 990

Ghoneim MA, Ashamallah A (1974) Further experience with the rectosigmoid bladder. Br J Urol 46: 511–519

Gilchrist RK, Merricks JW, Hamlin HH and Rieger IT (1950) Construction of substitute bladder and urethra. Surg Gynecol Obstet 90: 752–760

Goodwin WE, Scardino PT (1977) Ureterosigmoidostomy. J Urol 118: 169–174

Hammer E (1929) Cancer du colon sigmoide dix ans après implantation des urétères d'une vessie exstrophée. J Urol 28: 260–263

Hanley HG (1979) Bradshaw lecture on urinary diversion

Hansson HA, Kock NG, Norlen L, Philipson B, Trasti H, Ahren C (1978) Morphological observations in pedicled ileal grafts used for construction of continent reservoirs for urine. Scand J Urol Nephrol [Suppl] 49: 49–61

Harper JGM, Berman MH, Hertzberg AD, Lerman F, Brendler H (1954) Observations on the use of the cecum as a substitute urinary bladder. J Urol 71: 600–602

Heitz-Boyer M, Hovelacque A (1912) Creation d'une nouvelle vessie et un nouvel urètre. J Urol Nephrol 1: 237–258

Hinman F, Weyrauch HM (1936) A critical study of the different principles of surgery which have been used in uretero-intestinal implantation. Trans Am Assoc Genitourin Surg 29: 15

Hopewell J (1959) The hazards of uretero-intestinal anastomosis. Ann R Coll Surg Eng 24: 159–185

Irvine WT, Allan C, Webster DR (1956) Prevention of the late complications of ureterocolostomy by methods of faecal exclusion. Br J Surg 43: 650–658

Irvine WT, Yule JHB, Arnott DG, Peruma C (1960) Reduction in colonic absorption with reference to the chemical imbalance of ureterocolostomy. Proc R Soc Med 53: 1021–1027

Jacobs A (1967) A review of long-term results of ureterocolic anastomosis. Br J Urol 39: 670–675

Jacobs A, Stirling WB (1952) The late results of ureterocolic anastomosis. Br J Urol 24: 259–290

Kock NG, Nilson AE, Norlén L, Sundin T, Trasti H (1978a) Changes in renal parenchyma and the upper urinary tracts following urinary diversion via a continent ileum reservoir. An experimental study in dogs. Scand J Urol Nephrol [Suppl] 49: 11–22

Kock NG, Nilson AR, Norlén L, Sundin T, Trasti H (1978b) Urinary diversion via a continent ileum reservoir. Clinical experience. Scand J Urol Nephrol [Suppl] 49: 23–31

Kock NG, Myrvold HE, Nilsson LO, Ahrén C (1980) Construction of a stable nipple valve for the continent ileostomy. Ann Chir Gynecol 69: 132–143

Lapides J, Diokno AC, Lowe BS, Kalish MD (1974) Follow up on unsterile, intermittent self-catheterisation. J Urol 111: 184–187

Lapides J, Diokno AC, Gould FR, Lowe BS (1976) Further observations on self-catheterisation. J Urol 116: 169–171

Leadbetter WF (1951) Consideration of problems incident to the performance of ureteroenterostomy. Report of a technique. J Urol 65: 818–830

Leisinger HJ, Schauwecker H, Schmucki O, Hauri D, Mayor G, Säuberli H (1975) Continent ileal bladder. An experimental study in dogs. Eur Urol 1: 103–110

Leisinger HJ, Säuberli H, Schauwecker H, Mayor G (1976) Continent ileal bladder: First clinical experience. Eur Urol 2: 8–12

Lowsley OS, Johnson TH (1955) A new operation for creation of an artificial bladder with voluntary control of urine and feces. J Urol 73: 83–89

Madigan MR (1976) The continent ileostomy and the isolated ileal bladder. Ann R Coll Surg Eng 58: 62–69

Madigan MR (1978) Paper read to sections of Urology and Pathology. Royal Society of Medicine, 27th January, 1977

Mauclaire M (1895) De quelques essais de chirurgie experimentale applicables au traitement de l'exstrophie de la vessie et des anus contre nature complexes. Ann Mal Org Génito-urin 13: 1080–1086

Murphy LJT (1972) The history of urology. Thomas, Springfield, pp 288–332

Nesbit RM (1949) Ureterosigmoid anastomosis by direct elliptical connection: A preliminary report. J Urol 61: 728–734

Norlén L, Kock NG, Sundin T (1974) Cutaneous urinary diversion via a continent ileum reservoir. An experimental study in dogs. Lakaresällskapets Riksstämma, Stockholm

Perl JI (1949) Intussuscepted conical valve formation in jejunostomies. Surgery 25: 297–299

Riches EW (1967) A comparison of conduit and reservoir methods of urinary diversion. Br J Urol 39: 704–707

Rudick J, Schonholz S, Weber HN (1977) The gastric bladder: A continent reservoir for urinary diversion. Surgery 82: 1–8

Rudick J, Weber HN, Schonholz S, Corrigan M, Ciavarra V (1979) Evolution of a continent urostomy. Am Urol Assoc Meeting, New York

Rutishauser G (1977) Rectal bladder with dorsolateral intrasphincteric submucosal pull-through of the sigmoid colon in adult bladder cancer patients. Five years later. Eur Urol 3: 57–61

Schmidt, JD, Hawtrey CE, Flocks RH, Culp DA (1973) Complications, results and problems of ileal conduit diversion. J Urol 109: 210–216

Sinaiko ES (1960) Artificial bladder from gastric pouch. Surg Gynecol Obstet 111: 155–162

Smith GI, Hinman F Jr (1955) The intussuscepted ileal cystostomy. J Urol 73: 261–269

Stonington OG, Eiseman B (1956) Perineal sigmoidostomy in cases of total cystectomy. J Urol 76: 74–82

Sullivan H, Gilchrist RK, Merricks JW (1973) Ileocecal substitute bladder: Long-term follow up. J Urol 109: 43–45

Tacciuoli M, Laurenti C, Racheli T (1977) Sixteen years' experience with the Heitz Boyer-Hovelacque procedure for extrophy of the bladder. Br J Urol 49: 385–390

Trasti H (1978) Urinary diversion via a continent ileum reservoir. An experimental and clinical study. Scand J Urol Nephrol [Suppl] 49 (whole issue)

Tscholl R, Zingg E (1977) Der kontinente coeco-ileale Conduit. Die supravesikale Harnableitung. Huber, Bern, pp 146–154

Turner GG (1929) The treatment of congenital defects of the bladder and urethra by implantation of the ureters into the bowel: With a record of 17 personal cases. Br J Surg 17: 114–178

Turner-Warwick RT (1976) Urinary diversion. In: Blandy J (ed) Urology. Blackwell, Oxford, pp 1099–1122

Turner-Warwick RT, Ashken MH (1967) The functional results of partial, subtotal and total cystoplasty with special reference to ureterocaecocystoplasty, selective sphincterotomy and cystocystoplasty. Br J Urol 39: 3–12

Wallace DM (1966) Ureteric diversion using a conduit: A simplified technique. Br J Urol 38: 522–527

Whitaker RH, Pugh RCB, Dow D (1971) Colonic tumours following uretero-sigmoidostomy. Br J Urol 43: 562–575

Williams RE, Davenport TJ, Burkinshaw L, Hughes B (1967) Changes in whole-body potassium associated with uretero-intestinal anastomosis. Br J Urol 39: 676–680

Zingg E, Tscholl R (1977) Continent cecoileal conduit: Preliminary report. J Urol 118: 724–728

Subject Index

Renal Sonography

By F.S. Weill, E. Bihr, P. Rohmer, F. Zeltner
1981. 207 figures. XII, 134 pages
ISBN 3-540-10398-8

Diagnostic Imaging of the Kidney and Urinary Tract in Children

By A.R. Chrispin, I. Gordon, C. Hall, C. Metreweli
1980. 271 figures in 418 separate illustrations.
XVIII, 206 pages
(Current Diagnostic Pediatrics)
ISBN 3-540-09472-5

M.A. Meyers

Dynamic Radiology of the Abdomen

Normal and Pathologic Anatomy
With contribution on ultrasonography by E. Kazam
2nd edition 1982. 1038 figures (including 14 color
plates) Approx. 425 pages
ISBN 3-540-90629-0

Prostate Cancer

Editor: W. Duncan
1981. 68 figures, 67 tables. X, 190 pages
(Recent Results in Cancer Research, Volume 78)
ISBN 3-540-10676-6

Renal and Adrenal Tumors

Pathology, Radiology, Ultrasonography, Therapy,
Immunology
Editor: E. Löhr
Translated in Part from the German by
H.-U. Eickenberg
1979. 208 figures (14 in color) in 344 separate illu-
strations, 42 tables. XVIII, 372 pages
ISBN 3-540-09192-0

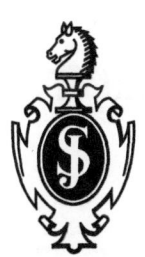

Springer-Verlag
Berlin
Heidelberg
NewYork

Idiopathic Hydronephrosis

Editors: P.H. O'Reilly, J.A. Gosling
Foreword by E.C. Edwards
1982. 87 figures. XII, 132 pages
ISBN 3-540-10937-4

The Ureter

Editor: H. Bergman
With 52 Contributors.
2nd edition. 1981. 760 figures. XVII, 780 pages
ISBN 3-540-90561-8

T. Mann, C. Lutwak-Mann

Male Reproductive Function and Semen

Themes and Trends in Physiology, Biochemistry and
Investigative Andrology.
1981. 46 figures. XIV, 495 pages
ISBN 3-540-10383-X

A.T.K. Cockett, K. Koshiba

Manual of Urologic Surgery

Illustrated by J. Takamoto
1979. 532 color illustrations
XVIII, 284 pages
(Comprehensive Manuals of Surgical Specialties)
ISBN 3-540-90423-9

Surgery of Female Incontinence

Editors: S.L. Stanton, E.A. Tanagho
With a Foreword by Sir John Dewhurst
1980. 199 figures, 17 tables. XVI, 203 pages
ISBN 3-540-10155-1

G.M. Bedbrook

The Care and Management of Spinal Cord Injuries

Foreword by R.W. Jackson
1981. 147 figures. XVI, 351 pages
ISBN 3-540-90494-8

Advances in Diagnostic Urology

Editor: C.C. Schulman
1981. 283 figures, 45 tables. XI, 339 pages
ISBN 3-540-10806-8

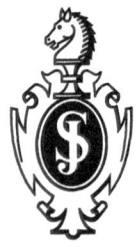

Springer-Verlag
Berlin
Heidelberg
New York